AIR FRYER Cookbook

Recipes to Lose Weight Rapidly on the Ketogenic Diet

(Treat Yourself With Oil-free Fried Food and Eat Healthy)

Henry Lathrop

Published by Alex Howard

© **Henry Lathrop**

All Rights Reserved

Air Fryer Cookbook: Recipes to Lose Weight Rapidly on the Ketogenic Diet (Treat Yourself With Oil-free Fried Food and Eat Healthy)

ISBN 978-1-989891-84-1

All rights reserved. No part of this guide may be reproduced in any form without permission in writing from the publisher except in the case of brief quotations embodied in critical articles or reviews.

Legal & Disclaimer

The information contained in this book is not designed to replace or take the place of any form of medicine or professional medical advice. The information in this book has been provided for educational and entertainment purposes only.

The information contained in this book has been compiled from sources deemed reliable, and it is accurate to the best of the Author's knowledge; however, the Author cannot guarantee its accuracy and validity and cannot be held liable for any errors or omissions. Changes are periodically made to this book. You must consult your doctor or get professional medical advice before using any of the suggested remedies, techniques, or information in this book.

Table of contents

Part 1 1
Introduction 2
Chapter 1: Tips before you get started 4
Chapter 2: 7 Days Ketogenic Diet Meal Plan 6
Chapter 3: My favorite Air Fry meals on a Keto Diet 12
Chapter 4: How an Air Fryer Complements a Keto Diet 14
Chapter 5: Why an Air Fryer is valuable for a Keto Diet 16
Chapter 6: Recipes 19
Breakfast 19
Herb Baked Eggs 19
Best Keto Cereal 20
Keto Grain-free Hemp Heart Porridge 21
Green Buttered Eggs - Keto and Low Carb 22
Avocado olive 23
Air Fried Chicken Wings 24
Keto broiled salmon with broccoli and cheddar 25
Cheddar Stuffed Meatballs 26
Lunch 27
Low-Carb Meat Pie 27
Italian Cabbage Stir-Fry 28
Spaghetti Squash Lasagna 29
Thin Crust Low Carb Pizza 31
Cheddar and Bacon BBQ Meatballs 32
Keto Air Fryer Fish Sticks 33
Fresh Air Fryer Pork Chops | Keto, Gluten Free 35

- Perfect Air Fryer Salmon 35
- Dinner 36
- Keto Swedish Meatballs (Grain-Free and Low Carb) ... 37
- Bangin' Coconut-Lime Skirt Steak 38
- Keto 5-Layer Mexican Dip Bowls 40
- Basic B Keto Dinner: Breaded Chicken, Whipped Cauliflower & Lemon Pepper Arugula Salad 41
- Low-Carb Spaghetti Squash Lasagna Recipe 43
- Air Fryer Parmesan Shrimp 44
- Low-Carb Herb-Marinated Air Fryer (Or Oven) Chicken Thighs 45
- Low Carb Keto Paleo Baked Chicken Nuggets in the Air Fryer 47
- Conclusion 49
- Part 2 50
- Who can benefit most from cooking with a fryer? 56
- How to preheat Air fryer? 58
- A step-by-step guide and a few things to keep in mind: 58
- RECIPES 62
- Avocado fries 62
- Roasted salmon with fennel salad 64
- Southern-Style Chicken 66
- Air fried vegetables 68
- Air-Fried Ham & Egg Toast Cups 69
- Air fryer pickle 72
- Parmesan chicken 73
- Manchurian Gobi 76
- Air Fryer Churros With Chocolate Sauce 79

Spicy roasted chicken breasts	82
Spanish frittata with potatoes and chorizo	84
Bourbon bacon burgers	86
Smoky sweet crunchy chickpeas	88
Strawberry tart	90
Air Fryer Garlic-Rosemary Brussels Sprouts	92
Smoked pork chops with raspberry	93
Breakfast style air fryer potato	95
Cinnamon rolls	98
Easy falafel recipe (GLUTEN FREE)	100
Doughnut	103
Air Fryer coconut shrimp and Apricot Sauce	105
Hash brown	107
Nashville hot chicken	109
Nashville Hot Sauce	111
Spicy kale chips	113
Lighten up Empanadas in an Air Fryer	115
Air Fryer Bourbon Bacon Cinnamon Rolls	117
Air fryer French Toast Sticks Recipe	119
Air Fryer Jalapeno Poppers	121
Peach pies	123
Air Fryer Chocolate Chip Oatmeal Cookies	124
Airfryer beetroot chips	126
Taco Bell crunch wraps	129
Homemade Croutons	131
Calzones	133
Air fryer fish and fries	135

- Pork taquitos 137
- Risotto balls 139
- Fried chicken wings 142
- Green tomato BLT 143
- Healthy fish finger sandwich 145
- Fried bananas S'mores 147
- Curried Sweet Potato Oven Fries with Creamy Cumin Ketchup 149
- Mexican corn in an air fryer 152
- Lemon biscuits 153
- Air fried potato recipe - potatoes with parsley and garlic ... 155
- Air fryer buffalo cauliflower 156
- Make delicious whole wheat pizza in an air fryer 158
- Lava cakes with peppermint 160
- Air Fryer Panko Breaded Chicken Parmesan with Marinara Sauce 162
- Roasted broccoli with cheese sauce 164
- TSO chicken 165
- Bourbon wings 168

Part 1

Introduction

This book contains steps and strategies on how to maintain a ketogenic diet. Not only that, I will also explain how you can use an air fryer to conveniently cook delicious ketogenic diet friendly meals.

Recently, the ketogenic diet has become a go-to diet for losing weight. Moreover, it has been known for aiding in managing some health conditions and has therefore received a lot of attention in the media.

If you are not familiar with this diet, you are probably asking yourself the following questions:
1. What is the ketogenic diet?
2. How does it work?
3. What is an air fryer?

The ketogenic diet is a high-fat, adequate-protein, low-carbohydrate diet. The diet forces the body to burn fats rather than carbohydrates. This causes a metabolic change in which the vital cell fuel source switches from carbohydrate-based fills (glucose) to fat energies and large ingestion system items called ketones. This is done over a metabolic procedure called ketogenesis, and a body state called ketosis. Ketosis is a usual metabolic pathway in which the body cells use ketones to make energy, instead of relying on sugar or carbohydrates.

Research is being conducted on ketosis as it relates to illnesses. Ketone bodies have positive effects on the human body and inspiring one's blood levels of ketone bodies is effective for some conditions because it improves the function of cell energy pathways and mitochondrial wellbeing. Ketogenic weight control plans are presently being used to treat medical conditions such as diabetes, epilepsy, autism, Alzheimer's and cancer.

The air fryer is a kitchen appliance that cooks by circulating hot air around the food using the convection mechanism. A mechanical fan circulates the hot air around the food at high speed, quickly cooking the food and producing a crispy layer. Compared to deep-frying, using an air fryer can reduce the amount of fat, calories and potentially harmful compounds in your food, making it a much better alternative to deep fryers.

Now you know the basics of what the keto diet is and how it works and also know what an air fryer does.

In the next chapter, you will get my most important tips and tricks before starting the actual "7 Days Ketogenic Diet Meal Plan".

Thereafter, I will tell you about some of the reasons to air fry on a keto diet. I have included some information, which I call a must know before starting your diet.

I am going to show you the main healthy, must-try ketogenic air fryer recipes in this cookbook which you are going to love. I have ensured they are easy and quick to follow even with a busy schedule.

Read this book, maintain your healthy ketogenic diet using an air fryer and enjoy all the benefits.

Thanks again for getting this book and happy cooking!

Chapter 1: Tips before you get started

One of the top tips I would like to share with you before you get started, is that you have the flexibility to swap the meal plans around. You may need to make small adjustments where you see fit. For instance, you can easily swap the lunch plan for dinner, breakfast for lunch, and so forth at any stage. You can also swap entire days if you like.

Also, remember that if you do not like certain ingredients in the meal plan, you can look over the recommended substitutions and choose ingredients that are more suitable for you. If you need to reduce fat, I would recommend to just reduce the amount of dairy and eggs. Also focus on added oils and fatty foods when making your adjustments. Do not stress over a surplus of protein, as it will not kick you out of ketosis. Moreover, the protein is actually what will keep the feeling of hunger under control.

Low-carb diets (below 30 grams of net carbs) are often said to be deficient in magnesium. I would therefore suggest for you to take magnesium supplements or to just add snacks that are high in magnesium to your diet. A great snack that is high in magnesium would be nuts like almonds, cashews or peanuts. Also, if you get any side effects such as "keto-flu", ensure you take in extra sodium. Personally, I use pink Himalayan salt for extra sodium. Please note that what is usually referred to as the "keto-flu" is when someone following a keto diet is experiencing all or some the following symptoms during their first week on the diet: fatigue, headache, dizziness, nausea, irritability and difficulty concentrating. Remember that the symptoms are only temporal, and you will feel better in no time.

Another tip I would like to share with you, is to always have some hard-boiled eggs in the fridge. These can be used in some recipes or for snacking in-between meals. Usually, you should not need any snacks between meals but if you do, ensure you have some keto-friendly snacks at hand. These could include snacks such as eggs, cheddar or nuts. The general rule is, if you do not feel hungry, don't eat, even if it means skipping dinner.

Please note that some recipes may be a little higher in fiber but that is fine. Fiber can indeed enable you to get in shape and lose weight in the right places. Body responses may differ, you should therefore be vigilant to know what works best for you.

Another great tip is, that if you are only cooking for yourself, you should freeze or refrigerate the rest of the servings or halve the recipes if you prefer. For instance, you can freeze half of the vegetarian Keto Lasagna for the following week.

A practical trick regarding the keto buns included in some of the meal plans is to prepare them in advance. I would suggest making the full recipe which will make around 10 buns. After preparing them, freeze to keep them crisp and defrost at room temperature the night before or in the oven just before serving.

To conclude, you should always discuss any dietary change with a health professional, especially if you have a health condition, for example diabetes or heart illness. There may need to be adjustments in accordance with the respective health condition or the medicine you are taking.

Chapter 2: 7 Days Ketogenic Diet Meal Plan

Let's get you introduced to the menu for one week on the ketogenic slim down plan.

Monday

Breakfast – 3 Egg Omelet with Spinach, Cheese and Sausage
Eggs should be categorized as one of the "superfoods" of our day, so eat eggs liberally. They are a very good source of high-quality protein and are packed with selenium, vitamin D, B6, B12 and minerals such as zinc, iron and copper. Another benefit of eating eggs is that they fill you up for hours, which is always a pro when it comes to diets.

Make an omelet with some cheddar, a breakfast hot-dog, and spinach. Spinach is an extraordinary source of magnesium and potassium. This should take you to just over 30g of protein for breakfast!

Incorporate some sea salt, and you have an important number of electrolytes that are key to keeping up essential nutrients and fighting off headaches. Get the details below.

Lunch – BLT Salad
Take 2-3 cups of lettuces, crumble in some bacon and dice a medium tomato.

Mix with a couple of tablespoons of mayo and toss after adding some hot sauce. My secret tip is to add some avocado pieces to lift potassium too!

I can guarantee that this will be tasty, filling, full of fiber, full of healthy fats and very easy to prepare. I realize the mayo sounds unusual as a dressing but trust me; it's a delicious combination!

Dinner – Baked Salmon with Asparagus

The great thing about salmon is that you can cook it quickly and with very minimal effort.

Create a quick sauce by mixing butter, lemon juice, cleaved garlic, some salt and pepper to enhance the natural taste of the salmon.

Sprinkle the sauce on more than 4-6 oz portions of fish, prepare at 450° F for 5 minutes for each ½ thickness of fish.

In another bowl, toss the asparagus in olive oil, salt and pepper, spread it out evenly on a cooking sheet, and roast on the grill at 450° F for 20 minutes.

This promises to be an easy dinner idea with potential leftovers for later. This meal is stacked with nutrition, protein, and healthy fats while keeping your carbs low.

Tuesday

Breakfast – Bacon and Eggs

A very easy dish to have at breakfast is 2-3 sautéed eggs and some bacon. Although this doesn't appear to be much, it's full of protein that will keep you full and strengthened to start off your day.

Lay your bacon strips on a single cooking sheet and prepare in the oven for 20 minutes at 40° F.

The result is the best bacon you have ever had, without sitting over a popping frying pan.

Lunch – Spinach Salad

You will rapidly find that salads are your best friend when in ketosis, and that for a good reason. Salads provide lots of nutrition to fill you up without weighing you down.

A bed of spinach with some red onion, bacon, a little tomato, and hot sauce vinaigrette is fast to put together and super tasty.

Add some protein such as maybe that leftover salmon from day 1 and voila you have a complete, large lunch.

To make the hot sauce vinaigrette, simply combine ½-cup olive oil, ¼-cup vinegar, hot sauce to taste and apply to salad. Ready to eat in a heartbeat!

Dinner – Cheese-Stuffed Bun less Burgers

Cook a few hamburger patties, and top one with cheddar and stack the other one on top. Don't forget to season the outside of the burger patties with a light sprinkling of salt and pepper, on both sides.

After they are cooked to your preference, place them on a plate, cover with veggies and low carb sauces and eat with a fork. Who needs the bun!

Wednesday

Breakfast – Eggies

You'll quickly find that eggs are essential for breakfast in low carb count plans. "Eggies" are the simple solution for a healthy breakfast.

Merely beat eight eggs in a bowl, incorporate cheddar and vegetables, and pour into muffin tins that have been fixed with a bit of bacon.

Cook at 350° F for 30 minutes, or until a toothpick stuck in the middle comes out dry. Store in baggies for breakfast for up to 5 days.

Lunch – Cottage Cheese, Walnuts and Hot Sauce

Hold on here, cottage cheese, walnuts and hot sauce? I know this sounds like an awful combination and I was doubtful too, but for a snappy and flavorful lunch you cannot go wrong here.

Then again, you could use cottage cheese and blueberries, if walnuts and hot sauce are not your thing.

Just mix them together and enjoy with a keto bun.

Dinner – Meatloaf

A better than average quality meatloaf needs meat and a binder, and luckily on keto, we have great choices for both. Using chopped mushrooms and onions as a binder rather than breadcrumbs, adds flavor and nutrients, and keeps carbs low. Add a veggie side, and you are prepared to go!

Thursday

Breakfast – Eggies

Lunch – Tuna Salad Lettuce Wraps
Making a tuna salad with low carb ingredients is easy, especially when you dice some fresh avocado into the salad. Use romaine lettuces to hold and eat the plate of mixed greens.

Dinner – Slaw Hash
Shred a cabbage head and cook with onions, ground beef, soy sauce, red pepper pieces, butter and garlic.
Sounds odd, but it tastes extraordinary. For more flavor, you could even use leftover chopped up meatloaf here if you have it.

Friday

Breakfast – Eggies or potentially Fat Coffee
Fat espresso is all the rage now and it is somewhat what it sounds like. Taking a nice quality espresso, and mixing it with 2 tbsp of grass-fed butter, 1-2 tablespoon of coconut oil, and stevia or whatever other zero-calorie sugar and flavors you like.
This coffee significantly lifts energy levels and suppresses hunger. It's also frothy and delicious!

Lunch – Spam Fries and Cole Slaw
If you spared some cabbage (uncooked) from last night's dinner, make a basic slaw using low carb ingredients, and

chop up some spam and cook in a frying pan for 20 minutes at 350° F. Serve with ranch or low carb ketchup!

Dinner – Tacos

Use your most preferred taco recipe, cook up some beef, and use romaine lettuces for shells. Incorporate some full-fat sour cream and cheddar, and you will never miss the tortillas.

Alert here, store-purchased taco seasoning is often full of carbs.

Saturday

Breakfast – Eggies

Lunch – Taco Salad

Take your remaining tacos and make a huge taco plate of mixed greens. Top with salsa, cream and some cheddar. Fat, protein, and veggies will fill you up all day!

Dinner – Pork Roast and Roasted Veggies

A nice pork roast rubbed down with cumin, salt and garlic, will give you delicious leftovers for days and the ingredients are very inexpensive.

Match the pork roast with some brussels sprouts, broccoli or cauliflower that has been roasted on the grill until brown, and you have a keto-style dinner!

Sunday

Breakfast – Avocado-Baked Eggs

Cut an avocado in two, take out the seed and split an egg into each avocado half. Bake until the egg is set. Voila, breakfast in the time it takes you to shower!

Lunch – Chicken and Hummus Lettuce Wraps

Chopped chicken, spread with hummus and wrapped with butter lettuce, is a quick lunch idea that gives you a protein punch without a huge number of calories.

Dinner – Philly Cheese steak Casserole

Using your remaining pork roast, mix in cut onions, peppers, cream cheddar, and shredded cheddar. Cook on the grill for 30 minutes at 350° F. Delightful, easy, and hearty, this meal is a crowd favorite, even for those that are not into low carb living!

Chapter 3: My favorite Air Fry meals on a Keto Diet

1. Keto-friendly veggies crisp up like a dream.

   I regularly make brussels sprouts that are impeccably fresh and done within only 10 minutes! They taste awesome and are so easy to make.
   Coat Brussels sprouts with olive oil, season to taste, and then cook in the air fryer for 10 minutes at 400° F. Halfway through cooking, stop and shake the basket to turn sprouts.

2. Make a keto-friendly breading with the air fryer.

   I made these crispy air fried pickles by making a breading out of ground parmesan cheddar and squashed pork rinds. First dredge pickles in almond flour, then in egg, then in the parmesan cheese and pork rind mixture. Place in an oiled air fryer basket in one single layer and spray the top with olive oil. Set the timer to 6 minutes at 370° F.

3. **Make PERFECT hard-boiled eggs without fail!**

   I love that there's no bubbling water needed for this fail proof method of cooking hard-boiled eggs. Simply put eggs in the fryer basket and set the clock to 16 minutes at 260°F. After the 16 minutes, give the eggs a chance to cool for a moment and then expel the shells under running water!

4. Air fried keto snacks rock!

   One easy satisfying snack idea is to air fry salami wrapped mozzarella cheddar sticks. Cut cheddar sticks into thirds, wrap each with a bit of salami and secure with a toothpick. Place in the air fryer and cook for 6 minutes at 360° F.

5. Kale chips have never been so crispy.

   If kale chips are your thing, it's good to know they turn out fantastic in the air fryer! To make these, separate around 3 cups of kale leaves from the stem. Toss in a little olive oil, salt and pepper, and then air fry for around 7 minutes at 370° F. Shake the basket half way through.

6. Make mess free bacon like a Boss.

Cook times will differ based on the thickness of the bacon used. Make traditional cut crispy bacon in only 8 minutes by air frying at 390° F. Thick sliced bacon may take more like 10-11 minutes or more to cook if you like really crispy bacon. Best of all, the grease drains to the base of the basket for easy cleanup!

7. Meat turns out DELICIOUS and juicy.

The air fryer goes beyond just tasty fries and snacks. I recently cooked some stunning burgers in the air fryer. Medium-sized patties can be cooked for around 9-10 minutes at 350 °F, or until cooked as desired.

8. Make crispy air fried wings with very little effort.

Put raw chicken wings in the air fryer basket, add salt and pepper to taste, and sprinkle with cooking oil. Set the clock to 30 minutes at 370° F. At 15 minutes turn them and spray the wings with cooking spray. When they are done, cover with wing sauce and enjoy! The texture and taste are PERFECT –crispy on the outside and juicy on the inside.

9. Leftovers have never tasted better.

Truly, you will never eat soggy leftovers again! I warmed up a leftover Keto Pizza the next day for only two or three minutes and it was perfectly crisp again!

Chapter 4: How an Air Fryer Complements a Keto Diet

Cooking meals for a low-carb or keto diet can be daunting and challenging. Certain ingredients are confined or beyond reach which can make it difficult to cook the meals you would like. An air fryer can definitely help to make things easier, if you are trying to follow a specific eating plan.

Here are some of the ways in which an air fryer can complement a low-carb diet:
- You can enjoy fried foods without the carbs
- Versatile cooking options keep things fun
- It makes cooking at home easier
- It saves time and space

Enjoying Fried Foods on a Low-Carb Diet

Fried foods are clearly seen as unhealthy and considered an unlikely part of a nutritious eating regimen. But air fryers turn that around. The progressive cooking technique allows you to achieve crispy, fried foods without having to use plenty of oil. This makes it possible to enjoy fried foods while staying on a diet. With an Air fryer, you can actually cut down the calories by more than 60% and even more when it comes to saturated fats.

Pick a low-carb breading alternative when frying foods for a keto diet. Nut flours are a great choice for low-carb breading. For some additional taste, try out finely chopped nuts as opposed to using nut flour. Toss foods in a monounsaturated cooking fat like avocado oil, coconut oil, or macadamia oil.

You can put some fried foods you had given up due to the keto diet back on the menu with an air fryer.

Here are a couple of great foods you can prepare with an air fryer:

- Eggplant chips
- Calamari rings
- Catfish
- Chicken pieces
- Mozzarella sticks
- Coconut chicken
- Shrimp
- Chicken wings
- Zucchini Parmesan chips
- Chicken tenders
- Crab cakes
- Tofu
- Onion rings
- Okra
- Parmesan cauliflower nibbles
- Kale chips

Chapter 5: Why an Air Fryer is valuable for a Keto Diet

Cook at Home Easily with an Air Fryer

Air fryers cook food by flowing hot air around the cooking basket, which cooks food much more rapidly than numerous conventional methods. This ensures that you get dinner on the table in no time, most especially in the wake of a difficult day at work. Simply take your ingredients, toss them all into the fryer, and let it work its magic.

Many fast foods, convenience foods, and prepared foods contain ingredients that ought to be avoided on a keto diet. Hence, cooking your own meals at home is an incredible method to control what exactly you are eating and also allows you to choose healthier food options as it gives you the chance you the chance to pick the exact ingredients.

Nevertheless, cooking at home on a regular basis is not convenient for everyone as the preparation takes additional time and at sometimes does not work with people's busy calendars. Fortunately, air fryers make it faster and more convenient to cook foods at home.

For instance, Frankfurters are one example of a great food to cook at home in your air fryer. Many store-bought sausages have fillers or different ingredients that make them not exactly perfect whilst on a low-carb diet. Picking your own meat and flavors, then cooking it in an air fryer will give you a yummy sausage that is easy to make and where you know the exact.

At the end of the day, having an efficient strategy for cooking delicious meals makes you more averse to get discouraged in your dieting journey.

Versatile Cooking Options

One thing that can be a genuine eating routine buster is eating the same foods repeatedly. Feeling stuck in a low-carb trench can prompt demotivation and can result in abandoning the diet. Air fryers are an incredible method to shake up a dull daily schedule. Due to versatile cooking options you can make a variety of incredible tasting low-carb foods.

You can roast, cook, broil, barbecue, and more in an air fryer. This one appliance makes preparing foods simple. Here are a few examples of some of the foods you can cook in an air fryer:

- Tofu
- Nuts
- Chicken
- Pork
- Fish
- Bacon
- Steak
- Vegetables
- Desserts

Obviously, within each category there is a scope of alternatives too. For instance, you can cook a rotisserie chicken or chicken fingers. All that makes the foods you can eat fun and enjoyable, even on a diet.

Air fryers also make reheating foods a snap. Have a go at getting huge portions of healthy, low-carb foods ready at the end of the week, then warm them throughout the week for quick dinners and side dishes. This is a great method to plan your meals without having to prepare foods from scratch every single day.

Desserts and Appetizers

It is rather difficult to entirely give up desserts whilst on a diet. An air fryer can prepare delightful low-carb dessert alternatives such as protein cakes, flourless chocolate cake, and low-carb doughnuts. With an air fryer, you can be totally creative and have a chance to explore the numerous possibilities of great recipes.

Appetizers are another fun category in which to get inventive with an air fryer. Chicken wings, vegetable chips, stuffed mushrooms, meatballs, and breaded shrimp are only a couple of tasty starters that are easy to cook in an air fryer. Consider cooking Shishito peppers when in the mood for something zesty. Hurl peppers with avocado oil, salt and pepper to taste, then cook in the air fryer for around ten minutes; complete with a splash of lime squeeze and ground asiago cheddar.

Chapter 6: Recipes

Breakfast

Herb Baked Eggs

Planning time: 10 minutes; Cooking time: 10 minutes; Serves: 4

Ingredients:

- 12 Large eggs
- 1/4 Cup heavy cream
- 2 Tablespoons parmesan cheese, grated
- 1 1/2 Tablespoons parsley, minced
- 1 Clove garlic, minced
- Salt and Pepper to taste
- 2 Tablespoons unsalted butter
- 1 Teaspoon oregano leaves, minced
- 1 Teaspoon thyme leaves, minced
- Toasted French bread or brioche for serving

Directions:

1. Preheat the grill pan for 5 minutes and place the oven rack 6 inch below the heat.
2. Combine the garlic, thyme, oregano, parsley, and parmesan cheese and set aside. Split three eggs into four small gratin dishes without breaking the yolks.
3. Place the four individual gratin dishes on a baking sheet. Put one tablespoon of cream and ½ tablespoon of butter in each dish and place in the oven for around 3 minutes, until hot and bubbly. Break three eggs into each gratin dish and sprinkle uniformly with the herb mix, and then sprinkle with salt and pepper. Place it back in the grill for 5-6 minutes,

until the whites of the eggs are cooked. Tip: Turn the baking sheet once if they are not cooking equally.

4.The eggs will keep on cooking after you have taken them out of the oven. Set them aside for 60 seconds and serve hot with toasted bread.

Best Keto Cereal

Planning time: 5 minutes; Cooking time: 8 minutes; Serves: 1 major bowl or 2 smaller dishes

Ingredients:

- 2 Cups Coconut/Almond/Flaxseed milk or Cream 18%, 35% etc. just keep in mind, the lower the carbs the better. For example, whole milk has more carbs than table cream.
- Dash of salt

Two of the following:

- 1/3 Cup toasted flaxseeds
- 1/2 cup shredded unsweetened coconut
- 1/3 Cup crushed walnut pieces
- Sweetener to taste
- 3-4 Teaspoon butter or ghee (omit to make vegan)
- 1/3 Cup crushed macadamia nut pieces

Directions:

1.In a metal pot on medium heat, soften the butter or ghee depending on which one you are using. If you prefer not to use butter or ghee, skip to stage 2. Toast the nuts and cracked coconut in a flame grill until wanted smoky taste.

2.Add the nuts and salt to the pot and mix rapidly for 1-2 minutes. Then add crushed coconut and keep blending. Ensure the bottom does not froth.

3. Incorporate 1 tablespoon of sugar to your pot with the nut/coconut mix.

4. Continue to blend and reduce the heat. You can serve it like this or let it cool down for 10 minutes.

Note: Notice how I mentioned just nuts and seeds high in omega-3. You can certainly use different nuts, for instance, you can cut up almonds, cashews etc. but I would strongly suggest adhering to the ones mentioned here, to get the full benefits. I need to also highlight the importance of the ratio of omega-3 to omega-6 to reliably check calories. Usually, we consume more omega-6, believing that its good fat, but not realizing that an inappropriate ratio of these two omegas can results in inflammation in the body.

Keto Grain-free Hemp Heart Porridge

Planning time: 2 minutes; Cooking time: 3 minutes; Serves: 1

Ingredients:

- 3/4 Teaspoon of pure vanilla extract
- Toppings
- 1 Tablespoon chia seeds
- 1/4 Cup crushed almonds or almond flour
- 1 Cup non-dairy milk
- 1/2 Cup Manitoba Harvest Hemp Hearts
- 1 Tablespoon xylitol or 5 drops alcohol-free stevia
- 3 Brazil nuts
- 1/2 Teaspoon ground cinnamon
- 2 Tablespoons freshly ground flax seed

Directions:

1. Add all ingredients but the ground almonds and garnishes to a little skillet. Mix until combined, then heat over medium heat, just until it starts to bubble.
2. Once foaming, blend once and leave to cook for another 1-2 minutes.
3. Take off from the heat, mix in almonds, and serve in a bowl. Top with your preferred toppings and you are ready to eat.

Note: I have not taken a try at making this keto recipe and eating it later. However, thinking of the ingredients there is a high possibility the porridge would get too sticky if not consumed right after cooking.

Regarding the nuts in this recipe, if you are unable to eat nuts due to allergies or just prefer not to add them, just exchange the ground almonds with sunflower seeds or pumpkin seeds.

Green Buttered Eggs - Keto and Low Carb

Planning time: 5 minutes; Cooking time: 12 minutes; Serves: 2 portions

Ingredients:

- 1/2 Cup fresh parsley, chopped
- 4 Organic eggs, ideally pastured
- 1 Teaspoon fresh thyme leaves
- 1/2 Cup fresh cilantro, chopped
- 2 Garlic cloves, peeled and finely chopped
- 1/4 Teaspoon ground cumin
- 1 Teaspoon coconut oil
- 2 Teaspoon organic butter, ideally pastured
- 1/4 Teaspoon ground cayenne
- 1/2 Teaspoon sea salt

Directions:
1. In a nonstick skillet (I use nontoxic stoneware) melt the butter and the coconut oil.
2. Add the chopped garlic cloves and cook on low heat for around 3 minutes or until the garlic starts sautéing.
3. Then incorporate the thyme and brown for around 30 seconds to a minute, do not let the garlic fume!
4. Add the cilantro and parsley to the dish and cook with moderate heat for around 3 minutes, until brown.
5. Put the eggs into a bowl, splitting them straight in, being mindful so as not to break the yolk.
6. Cover the pot and lower the heat.
7. Cook for around 4-6 minutes until yolks are set but still soft inside. If you prefer your yolks runny, then cook for just 3-4 minutes.
9. Now, serve immediately. Can be combined with some breakfast wiener and/or grain saltines.

Avocado olive

Planning time: 5 minutes; Cooking time: 6 minutes; Serves: 4

Ingredients:
- 1 Teaspoon Herbs De Provence
- 2 Teaspoon MCT Oil (Medium-chain triglyceride)
- 10 Kalamata olives, pitted
- 1/2 Teaspoon sea salt
- 2 Teaspoon organic butter
- 4 Pastured or organic eggs
- 2 oz. Full-fat Brie Cheese
- 1 Avocado

Directions:

1. In a big bowl, whisk the eggs with the MCT oils, the herbs de Provence, the olives and the salt until foamy.
2. Split, strip and slice the avocado and then cut into thick pieces.
3. In a skillet beat the butter on high heat until frothy, then add the avocado and mix with the butter.
4. Take out with a spatula and set aside.
5. Still, on high heat add the egg blend into the skillet.
6. Cut the brie into thin slices and place it in the egg mix.
7. Now, cover the skillet and cook for around 3 minutes or until the base of the frittata is brown.
8. Flip the frittata and cook for an additional 2 minutes.
9. Serve it hot on a plate and garnished with the avocado.

Air Fried Chicken Wings

Planning time: 3 minutes; Cooking time: 30 minutes; Serves: 4

Ingredients:

- 2 Pounds organic chicken wings
- Fine grain sea salt

Directions:

1. Preheat the air fryer mode to 400° F.

2. Pat the chicken wings dry with a paper towel. Place onto baking paper and sprinkle with fine grain ocean salt.

3. Place into the air fryer for 30 minutes or until the point when chicken wings are cooked and crispy.

Tip: Serve with ranch dressing. Personally, I use Primal Kitchen farm, which tastes great and is also dairy free!

Keto broiled salmon with broccoli and cheddar

Planning time: 5 minutes; Cooking time: 20 minutes; Serves: 2

Ingredients:

- 1 lb Broccoli
- 1½ lbs Salmon
- 3 oz. Butter
- Salt and pepper
- 5 oz. Grated cheddar cheese
- 1 Lime (optional)

Directions:

1. Preheat the oven to 400° F (200°C).
2. Cut the broccoli into smaller florets and let stew in slightly salted water for 2-3 minutes. Ensure the broccoli keeps up its chewy texture and color. Drain the broccoli and dispose of the water. Set aside for a moment or two and allow the steam to disappear.
3. Place the broccoli into a well-greased cooking dish. Add butter and pepper to taste.
4. Sprinkle cheddar over the broccoli and cook in the oven for 15-20 minutes or until the cheddar turns into a golden color.
5. In the meantime, season the salmon with salt and pepper and fry in butter, a couple of minutes on each side. The lime can be served raw or a splash added to the Salmon. This recipe can also be cooked on an outdoor grill.

Note:

Remember, you can be flexible and substitute the broccoli for different vegetables, with practically zero change in the amount of carbs in the dish. For example, I can see this recipe going great with brussels sprouts, green beans or asparagus.

In addition to that, if you want to use another type of fish, I would suggest other greasy fishes. Here I would recommend trout or mackerel, but you can also go with white fish if you wish.

If you do not like cheddar, you can use a blend of different cheeses. I can already see that half mozzarella and half parmesan would also make a delicious combination!

Cheddar Stuffed Meatballs

Planning time: 10 minutes; Cooking time: 20 minutes; Serves: 6

These low carb cheddar stuffed meatballs have awesome flavor and a mushy texture!

Ingredients:

- 2 Eggs
- 20 oz. Ground beef
- 1 Teaspoon Italian seasoning
- Salt and pepper
- 1/4 Cup grated Parmesan
- 10 oz. Ground pork
- 3 Cheese string sticks

Directions:

1. Preheat the oven to 375° F.
2. In a huge bowl mix the pork, beef, egg, parmesan and seasonings.
3. Cut the cheddar strings into small pieces.

4. Take a handful of the meat blend, form into a ball and press a piece of the cheddar string into the center. Seal the meat tightly around the cheese. This recipe will make for roughly 24 meatballs.

5. Place the meatballs onto baking paper and cook for 15-20 minutes until the meat is cooked and the cheddar has softened.

Lunch

Low-Carb Meat Pie

Planning time: 15 minutes; Cooking time: 15 minutes; Serves: 6

Ingredients:

- 2 Tablespoons butter or olive oil
- 1 1/3 lbs Ground beef or ground lamb
- 3 Tablespoons coconut oil
- Salt and pepper
- 1 Tablespoon dried oregano or dried basil
- 4 Tablespoons tomato paste or ajvar relish
- 1/2 Cup water
- Pie crust
- 3/4 Cup almond flour
- 1/4 Cup sesame seeds
- 1/4 Cup coconut flour
- 1 Egg
- 1/4 Cup water
- 1 Onion, finely chopped
- 1 Garlic clove, finely chopped
- Topping
- 8 oz. cottage cheese
- 7 oz. Shredded cheese

- 1 Tablespoon ground psyllium husk powder
- 1 Teaspoon baking powder

Directions:

1. Fry onion and garlic in oil on medium heat for several minutes, until the onion is soft. Add the ground meat and keep frying. Then add salt, pepper, and incorporate the oregano or dried basil.
2. Add tomato paste, pesto or ajvar relish. Incorporate some water, lower the heat and let stew for approximately 20 additional minutes while you are making the pie mix.
3. Preheat the oven to 350° F (175°C).
4. Blend all the batter ingredients in a food processor for a few minutes until the mix changes into a ball. If you do not have a food processor, you can also use a fork to mix.
5. Wrap the cooked beef with a bit of greased baking paper (around 10 inch in measurement) to make it easier to remove the pie when it is set. Spread the batter into the shape and fold up the edges. Use a spatula or all around greased fingers.
6. Pre-bake the pie for 10-15 minutes. Remove it from the oven and place the meat in the outside layer. Blend curds, cheddar, and extra topping.
7. Bake for 15 minutes on a lower rack or until the pie has turned golden brown.
8. This dish goes great with a small side salad and dressing.

Italian Cabbage Stir-Fry

Planning time: 10 minutes; Cooking time: 10 minutes; Serves: 4

Ingredients:

- 1 Teaspoon onion powder

- 1/4 Teaspoon pepper
- 5 oz. Butter
- 1 1/3 Pounds ground beef
- 1/2 Cup fresh basil
- 1 Tablespoon white wine vinegar
- 1 Teaspoon salt
- 2 Garlic cloves, finely chopped
- 3 oz. Leeks, thinly sliced
- 1 Tablespoon tomato paste
- 1 2/3 lbs Green cabbage
- 1 Cup mayonnaise or sour cream, for serving

Directions:

1. Shred the green cabbage finely with a cheddar slicer, sharp knife or in a food processor.
2. Broil the cabbage in butter (or extra olive oil) on a large grill or in a wok on medium heat for around 10 minutes.
3. **Include vinegar, salt, onion powder, and pepper. Blend and sear for 2-3 minutes, or until all is combined. Serve sautéed cabbage to a bowl.**
4. Heat remains of the butter or oil on the grill or in wok and include the garlic and leeks. Sauté for a few minutes.
5. Include meat and keep stirring until cooked through.
6. Include tomato paste and blend well. Lower the heat a little and include cabbage and basil. Mix until cooked through.
7. Add seasoning and serve with a dab of cream or mayonnaise and maybe even a plate of mixed greens.

Spaghetti Squash Lasagna

Planning time: 5 minutes; Cooking time: 6 minutes; Serves: 2

Ingredients:

- 2 Cloves of minced garlic (equivalent to 1 teaspoon)
- 1 Egg

- 1 Teaspoon chili powder
- 5 Grinds of sea salt
- 2 1/2 Cups spaghetti squash
- 1 Teaspoon crushed red pepper flakes
- 1 Cup grated parmesan cheese
- 1 lb Organic ground beef, ideally grass fed
- 1/2 Teaspoon basil
- 3 Grinds of fresh pepper
- 2 Cups mozzarella cheese, shredded
- 1/2 Teaspoon oregano
- 3/4 Jar pasta sauce, average-sized

Directions:

1. Preheat oven to 400° F (200°C). Cut spaghetti squash down the middle and scoop out seeds and filaments. Season with salt and dark pepper; cook on a baking sheet for around 60 minutes, or more if needed. If you would prefer to use the microwave, cut squash down the middle, scoop out seeds and filaments, place on a microwave safe dish and cover. Microwave 8-9 minutes or until delicate.

2. In a small bowl, combine the ricotta, cheddar, parmesan cheddar and parsley.

3. In a large sauté skillet, heat oil and include onions and garlic. Sauté on medium-low heat for around 3-4 minutes. Include the sausage and cook, separate into smaller pieces until seared and cooked through. When cooked, include the sliced tomatoes, add salt and pepper to taste. Reduce heat to low and stew 20-30 minutes, including fresh basil at the end.

4. **When spaghetti squash is cooked, let it cool for around 10 minutes keeping the oven on. If you used the microwave, preheat the oven to 400° F (200°C) now.**

5. When the spaghetti squash is cool enough, use a fork to remove flesh, which will turn out in spaghetti looking strands. Remember to save the shells. Reduce the squash on a paper towel to extract any excess fluid. Toss with half of the sauce,

place the spaghetti squash into the shells and place on a baking sheet.

6. Top each with sauce, 1 scoop ricotta- cheddar blend and a little mozzarella cheddar.

7. Bake in the oven for 20-30 minutes or until everything is hot and the cheddar has melted.

8. If you are short on time, you can brown the sausage and include a container of spaghetti sauce as opposed to making and braising the sauce.

9. Make the receipt veggie friendly by leaving out the sausage.

Thin Crust Low Carb Pizza

Planning time: 2 minutes; Cooking time: 6 minutes; Serves: 4

Ingredients:

- 2 oz. cheese per pita (Low-moisture mozzarella is a great base, then add others of your choosing)
- Roasted red peppers
- Olives, artichokes, pesto
- Few tablespoons tomato sauce, enough to cover pita (my favorite is Classico which has lots of flavor)
- Chili flakes - dash
- Optional mix-Ins
- Ground black pepper - dash
- Garlic powder - dash
- Joseph's Low-Carb Pita Bread (choose desired quantity and size)
- Bacon
- Spinach
- Any other ingredients, customize it to whatever dietary need or taste you enjoy e.g. Pepperoni, salami, prosciutto, roast beef, ham, pineapple, mango, avocado, rooster sauce.

Directions:

1. Preheat oven to a toasty 450° F (230°C)
2. Either brush Josephs low carb pita bread with oil or spray both sides with cooking spray.
3. Place on grill for 1- 2 minutes and toast.
4. Take from grill and add the sauce.
5. Add cheeses (mozzarella first)
6. Add garnishes of your choice
7. Rub with some olive oil and toast for 1-2 minutes at 450° F (230°C) until crispy.
8. Bake for an extra 3-6 minutes to soften the cheddar.

Cheddar and Bacon BBQ Meatballs

Planning time: 6 minutes; Cooking time: 10 minutes; Serves: 5

Ingredients:

- 3/4 Teaspoon garlic Powder
- 4 Slices Bacon
- 3/4 Cup Cheddar Cheese
- 3/4 Cup Crushed Pork Rinds (BBQ Flavor if you have it)
- 3/4 Teaspoon Cumin
- 3/4 Teaspoon Salt
- 1 Large Egg
- 1.5 Pounds (93/7) ground Beef
- 3/4 Teaspoon Pepper
- BBQ sauce of your choice

Directions:

1. Put the pork skins into a Ziploc bag and beat with a meat tenderizer.

2.In a dish, mix your ground beef, egg, salt, pepper, cumin, and garlic powder.
3.Add your pork skin pieces and mix well.
4.Make a bit of an opening in the meat, add your cheddar and mix.
5.Cut your 4 cuts of bacon into thin strips. The easiest way is to use scissors.
Tip: If you intend to use a knife, put your bacon in the fridge for 20 minutes before cutting it.
6.Add your bacon to a hot dish and let it cook.
8.Place your bacon aside on a paper towel. Keep the dish with the bacon fat in it – as you will use it to cook the meatballs!
9.Once your bacon has cooled a bit, add it to the meat mix.
10.Usually, this recipe will make around 20-25 meatballs of a great size. Take the meatballs out of the oven and put them aside.
11.Add about half of them to the dish to start cooking.
12.Let them brown on one side and then flip them over.
13.Allow them to keep cooking, turning them as required.
14. Take them from the dish when they are still semi-raw on the inside.
15.Reduce the heat to low and cover the dish with a top. Let it cook.
16. Set the meatballs aside and let them rest for around 5 minutes.
17.Serve them topped with your BBQ sauce, (approximately 4-5 meatballs for each individual).

Keto Air Fryer Fish Sticks

Planning time: 10 minutes; Cooking time: 10 minutes; Serves: 4

Crispy breaded keto fish sticks! This air fryer fish recipe is so simple and a total family pleaser.

Calories: 263 kcal

Ingredients:

- 1 1/2 Cups pork rind panko such as Pork King Good
- 3/4 Teaspoon Cajun seasoning
- 1/4 Cup mayonnaise
- 1 lb White fish such as cod
- 2 Tablespoon water
- 2 Tablespoon Dijon mustard
- Salt and pepper to taste

Directions:

1. Spray the air fryer rack with non-stick cooking spray (I use avocado oil).
2. Pat the fish dry and cut into sticks around 1 inch by 2 inches wide. How you can cut it will depend on what fish you use and how thick and wide it is.
3. In a small shallow bowl, whisk together the mayo, mustard, and water. In another shallow bowl, whisk together the pork skins and Cajun seasoning. Add salt and pepper to taste. Both the pork skins and seasoning could have a fair amount of salt so make sure to dip a finger in to taste how salty it is.
4. Working with one bit of fish at a time, dunk into the mayo mixture to coat and then tap off the excess. Thereafter, dip into the pork skin mixture to coat. Place on the air fryer rack.
5. Set to air fry at 400°F (200°C) and fry for 5 minutes, then flip the fish sticks with tongs and bake for an extra 5 minutes. Serve quickly.

Note:

Even if you do not have an air fryer, you can still make these tasty keto fish sticks. Just preheat your oven to 425°F (218°C) and add a few tablespoons of oil to a rimmed sheet skillet. Place the sheet pan in the oven while it preheats.

Place the covered fish sticks on the sheet pan and bake for 5 minutes, then flip over and bake for another 5 minutes.

Fresh Air Fryer Pork Chops | Keto, Gluten Free

Planning time: 5 minutes; Cooking time: 12 minutes; Serves: 6

Calories: 222 kcal, 11g fat, 2g carbs, 1g fiber, 26g protein. 1 net carb!

Ingredients:

- 1 Teaspoon garlic powder
- 1/3 Cup Almond Flour
- 1 Teaspoon Paprika
- 1 Teaspoon Tony Chachere's Creole Seasoning
- 1/4 Cup grated Parmesan cheese
- 1 1/2 lb Boneless pork chops

Directions:

1. Preheat your air fryer to 360° F (180°C)
2. Meanwhile, mix all ingredients except the pork chops in a big zip lock bag.
3. **Place the pork chops into the bag, seal it and then shake to coat the pork.**
4. **Remove from the bag and then place in the air fryer in a single layer. Cook for 8-12 minutes depending on the thickness of your pork chops.**

Perfect Air Fryer Salmon

Planning time: 10 minutes; Cooking time: 15 minutes; Serves: 2

Ingredients:

- 2 Salmon fillets with comparable thickness, mine were 1-1/1 2-inches thick
- Generously seasoned with salt and coarse black pepper
- 2 Teaspoons avocado oil or olive oil
- 2 Teaspoons paprika
- Lemon wedges

Directions:

1. Remove any bones from your salmon and let it sit for 60 minutes. Rub each filet with olive oil and season with paprika, salt and pepper.
2. Place filets in the basket of the air fryer. Set air fryer to 390° F (190°C) for 7 minutes for 1-1/2-inch filets.
3. **After the 7 minutes, open the basket and check filets with a fork to ensure they are done.**
4. **Time for cooking will differ for salmon based on the temperature of the fish and the width of your filets. I would recommend making a habit of setting your air fryer to a bit less time than you would expect until you become more used to the timing.**

Note:

One of the delights of air fryers is that it is so easy to pop something back in for a moment if you want it cooked longer. You can also open it while it is still cooking to ensure it is not overdone. Like mentioned above, I usually set my timer to somewhat less time, so I can keep an eye on how things are tagging along and avoid overcooking meals.

Dinner

Keto Swedish Meatballs (Grain-Free and Low Carb)

Planning time: 10 minutes; Cooking time: 30 minutes; Serves: 4

Ingredients:

- 1/2 Teaspoon ground nutmeg
- 1 Cup shredded mild Cheddar cheese
- Cups heavy whipping cream
- 1 Large egg
- 1 Tablespoon water
- 1/4 Cup diced onions
- Cups chicken broth
- 2 lbs Ground meatloaf mixture or 1 lb ground beef and 1lb ground pork
- 1 Tablespoon Dijon mustard
- 1/4 Teaspoon allspice
- 4 Tablespoons salted butter
- 1 Tablespoon Worcestershire sauce

Directions:

1. Preheat oven to 400° F (200°C) and preheat a slow cooker to low.
2. Line a broad baking tray with baking paper.
3. In a big bowl, combine ground meat, cheddar, egg, onion, water, nutmeg and allspice.
4. Roll the mix into 1.5-inch meatballs and place them on the lined dish (you may require two depending on how big your dish is)
5. Bake for around 20 minutes

6. Meanwhile, in a little skillet, heat the butter, chicken stock, and cream over medium heat.
7. Once it starts to stew, reduce the heat to low and keep stewing for around 20 minutes. Remember to keep stirring.
8. Now stir in the mustard and Worcestershire sauce.
9. Pour the sauce into a moderately sized cooker and add the meatballs when they are ready.
10. Cook on low heat for around 2 hours so the meatballs can marinate.
11. Stir every half hour or thereabouts, covering all the meatballs. Do not cook them in the moderate cooker for longer than two hours, or the sauce may start to separate.

Bangin' Coconut-Lime Skirt Steak

Planning time: 10 minutes; Cooking time: 30 minutes; Serves: 4

Ingredients:

- 1 Teaspoon grated fresh ginger
- Zest of one lime
- 2 Tablespoons freshly squeezed lime juice from one lime
- 1/2 Cup coconut oil, melted
- 3/4 Teaspoon sea salt
- 1 Tablespoon minced garlic
- 1 Teaspoon red pepper flakes (depending on how much spice you would prefer)
- 2 lb Grass fed skirt steak (can be cut into sections)

Directions:

1. In a large bowl, mix the coconut oil, lime juice, lime zest, garlic, ginger, red pepper flakes and salt.

2.Add the steak and rub with the marinade (the coconut oil will freeze after you are done which is normal).
3.Let meat marinate for around 20 minutes at room temperature.
4.Transfer steak to a big skillet set over medium-high heat. If a portion of your marinade is still stuck to the bowl, spoon it out into the pan to cook the steak.
5.Sear the steak on both sides for approximately 4-5 minutes on each side or until it's cooked to your liking.
6.Cut and serve!

Keto 5-Layer Mexican Dip Bowls

Planning time: 10 minutes; Cooking time: 45 minutes; Serves: 18

Ingredients:

For the guac

- 1 Small tomato, or 6 cherry tomatoes, seeded and chopped
- 1 Teaspoon minced garlic
- 1/4 Cup fresh cilantro, chopped
- 1/2 Teaspoon sea salt
- 2 Ripe avocados, peeled, pitted, and cut into chunks
- 1 Tablespoon freshly squeezed lime juice (or out of a bottle)
- 1/4 Cup white onion, chopped

For the beef

- 1/4 Cup taco seasoning (preferably a low-carb and sugar-free one)
- 2 Cups shredded lettuce
- 2 Cups shredded cheddar cheese
- 2 lbs Grass fed ground beef
- 2 Cups organic sour cream
- 1/2 Cup water
- Cayenne pepper sauce (to taste)

Directions:

1. In a medium bowl, mash together avocado, lime juice, cilantro, onion, tomato, garlic, and salt.

2. Cover the guac and refrigerate while you cook the meat.
3. In a medium skillet, cook the ground beef over medium heat for around 10 minutes.
4. Stir in the water and taco seasoning. Reduce the heat and cook for 10 minutes.
5. Transfer the beef into four little dishes.
6. Top with sour cream, then guacamole, then the lettuces, then the cheddar. Finally, sprinkle some cayenne pepper over the top to your preference.

Basic B Keto Dinner: Breaded Chicken, Whipped Cauliflower & Lemon Pepper Arugula Salad

Planning time: 15 minutes; Cooking time: 45 minutes; Serves: 3

Ingredients:

For the breaded chicken:

- 1 Bag of 5 Perdue Perfect Portions Boneless, Skinless Chicken Breast (Italian Style)
- 3 oz. Crushed pork rinds
- 1/2 Cup grated parmesan cheese
- 1/2 Tablespoon Italian seasoning
- 1/2 Teaspoon garlic salt

For the buttery cauliflower mash:

- 1 Bag (16 oz.) Green Giant Fresh Cauliflower Crumbles (or 4 cups chopped cauliflower, steamed)
- 2 Tablespoons ghee (or 2 tablespoons salted butter)
- 2 Tablespoons butter (if you don't have ghee, just use 4 tbsp butter)
- 1/2 Cup heavy cream
- 1/4 Cup shredded parmesan cheese
- A pinch of garlic salt
- A pinch of seasoning salt (like Adobo)
- A bit of pepper to taste

For the salad:

- 1 Tablespoon high-quality extra virgin olive oil
- 1/2 Tablespoon fresh lemon juice
- 3 Cups baby arugula
- A couple of fresh grinds of sea salt and pepper

Directions:

For the chicken

1. Preheat the oven to 375° C.
2. Set up a wire roasting rack over a backing sheet (this is so the chicken does not sit on the bottom and get soggy – you can also use a backing rack if it is oven-friendly).
3. **On a plate, mix the crushed pork rinds, grated parmesan, Italian seasoning and garlic salt.**
4. Put a breast of chicken into the blend, cover completely and set on the rack.
5. When done, put in the oven for 20 minutes, or until baked to around 165 degrees, then turn the oven off and let sit in to keep cooking.

For the buttery cauliflower mash

1. In a blender, combine everything except for the cauliflower. Do not to blend yet.
2. Chop cauliflower and microwave for 1 minute. Leave the top open for 4 minutes. Then microwave for another minute.
3. **Add steamed cauliflower to a blender, and blend to the consistency you like.**

For the serving of mixed greens
   In a bowl, mix all ingredients until each leaf is coated.

For plating
   Once everything is done, just plate your chicken, whipped cauliflower and arugula salad between 4 dishes.
   Tip: I always like to sprinkle some parmesan cheese over the greens and add a grind of fresh pepper over the cauliflower. In addition to that, when I feel particularly adventurous, I like to serve this dish with a side of Dijon mustard as a dip.

Low-Carb Spaghetti Squash Lasagna Recipe

Planning time: 30 minutes; Cooking time: 20 minutes; Serves: 6

Ingredients:
- 1/2 Teaspoon basil
- 3/4 Average-sized jar pasta/tomato sauce
- 1 Teaspoon crushed red pepper flakes
- 5 Grinds of sea salt
- 3 Grinds of fresh pepper
- 2 1/2 Cups spaghetti squash (roasted for an hour at 350°C)

- 2 Cloves of minced garlic
- 1/2 Teaspoon oregano
- 1 Egg
- 1 lb Organic grass-fed ground beef
- 1 Cup grated parmesan cheese
- 1 Teaspoon chili powder
- 2 Cups shredded mozzarella cheese

Directions:

1. Roast your spaghetti squash in the oven for an hour at 350° F or cook it in the microwave for 20 minutes. Allow it to sit for 5 minutes afterward.
2. Heat sauce and add red pepper flakes. Allow to stew with cover on.
3. Blend meatball ingredients in a bowl and roll into quarter-sized smaller than normal meatballs.
4. Heat a big frying skillet on medium heat with a tablespoon of ghee, butter or oil.
5. Cook meatballs in the frying dish and cover. Flip at approx. 3-5 minutes.
6. When the meatballs are cooked through, use a spoon to add them (without the grease) into the sauce.
7. In the meantime, chop the squash down the center and scrape 2 ½ measures of spaghetti squash (empty seeds and guts first). Set aside.
8. In a little bread dish (tall and thin), layer sauce, squash, meatballs, sauce, mozzarella, squash, meatballs, sauce, mozzarella.

Air Fryer Parmesan Shrimp

Planning time: 20 minutes; Cooking time: 20 minutes; Serves: 2

Simple and tasty garlic and parmesan air-fried shrimp, prepared in 20 minutes!

Ingredients:
- 1 Teaspoon pepper
- 1/2 Teaspoon oregano
- 1 Teaspoon onion powder
- 2 Tablespoons olive oil
- 1 Teaspoon basil
- 2 Pounds jumbo cooked shrimp, peeled and deveined
- 4 Garlic cloves, minced
- 2/3 Cup parmesan cheese, grated
- 1 Lemon, quartered

Directions:
1. In a large bowl, mix garlic, parmesan cheddar, pepper, oregano, basil, onion powder and olive oil.
2. Gently toss shrimp in mixture until evenly covered.
3. Spray air fryer basket with non-stick spray and place shrimp in basket.
4. Cook at 330° F for 20 minutes or until seasoning on shrimp is brown and crispy.
5. Squeeze the lemon over the shrimp before serving.

Notes:
If using an oven, prepare at 200°C degrees for 8-10 minutes.

Low-Carb Herb-Marinated Air Fryer (Or Oven) Chicken Thighs

Planning time: 15 minutes; Cooking time: 20-35 minutes; Serves: 6-10

Low-Carb Herb-Marinated Air Fryer (or Oven) Chicken Thighs are an inexpensive, fast and tasty idea for a low-carb dinner.

Ingredients:

- 1/2 Teaspoon onion powder
- 1/2 Teaspoon dried sage
- 1/2 Teaspoon dried oregano
- 1 Teaspoon dried basil
- 2 Teaspoons lemon juice
- 2 Teaspoons garlic powder
- 1 Teaspoon Spike seasoning or alternatively any all-purpose herb blend
- 6-10 Bone-in, skin-on chicken thighs
- 1/4 Cup olive oil
- 1/4 Teaspoon black pepper

Directions:

1. Trim off some of the skin and the fat from the chicken thighs (I normally use kitchen shears to trim the chicken)
2. Mix together olive oil, lemon juice, garlic powder, Spike seasoning, dried basil, dried oregano, onion powder, dried sage, and dark pepper to make the marinade.
3. Put chicken thighs in a Ziploc bag or plastic dish with a snap-tight lid, add the marinade and let the chicken marinate in the fridge for around 6 hours, or all day while you are at work.
4. When you are ready to cook, drain the chicken in a strainer.
5. Arrange chicken top-side down all around the air fryer basket or on a baking rack and let the chicken come to room temperature while you preheat the air fryer to 360° F (185°C) or if you are using the oven preheat it to 400° F (200°C).
6. **To Cook in Air Fryer:** Cook chicken top-side down in the pre-heated air fryer for 8 minutes. Then turn the chicken thighs over and cook for around 10-12 minutes. Following

the 6 minutes, check that the chicken is all around crispy and the internal temperature is at 165° F (75°C).

To Cook in the Oven: Cook chicken top-side down in the preheated oven for 10 minutes. Then turn chicken pieces over and cook around 25 minutes longer or until the chicken is sautéed and the skin is crispy. Serve hot.

Low Carb Keto Paleo Baked Chicken Nuggets in the Air Fryer

Planning time: 10 minutes; Cooking time: 15 minutes; Serves: 4

Calories 286 kcal

These Low Carb Keto Paleo Baked Chicken Nuggets have an Asian twist to them! A solid, gluten free, family-accommodating weeknight dinner!

Ingredients:

- 1 Pound Free-range boneless, skinless chicken breast
- 1/2 Teaspoon ground ginger
- 4 Egg whites
- 6 Tablespoons toasted sesame seeds
- A pinch of sea salt
- 1 Teaspoon sesame oil
- 1/4 Cup coconut flour
- Cooking spray of choice

For the dip:

- 2 Tablespoons natural creamy almond butter
- 2 Teaspoons rice vinegar
- 1 Teaspoon sriracha to taste
- 4 Teaspoons coconut aminos (or GF soy sauce)
- 1 Tablespoon water

- 1/2 Teaspoon ground ginger
- 1/2 Teaspoon monk fruit

Directions:

1. Preheat you air fryer to 400° F for 10 minutes.
2. While the air fryer warms, cut the chicken into chunks (around 1-inch pieces) get them dry and place them in a bowl. Toss in salt and sesame oil until fully covered.
3. Place the coconut flour and ground ginger in a Ziploc sack and shake. Add the chicken and shake again until covered.
4. Place the egg whites in a large bowl and add the chicken strips, shake until they are all around covered in the egg.
5. Place the sesame seeds in a Ziploc bag. Shake any extra egg off the chicken and add the nuggets into the pack, shake until covered all around.
6. Spray the air fryer basket with cooking spray. Place the pieces into the basket; making sure not to crowd them or they will not get crispy.
7. Cook for 6 minutes. Flip every piece again and spray with cooking spray. Then, cook an extra 5-6 minutes until crispy and juicy.
8. While the nuggets cook, mix all the sauce ingredients together in a medium bowl until smooth.
9. Serve the nuggets with the dip and enjoy!

Conclusion

People are always looking for appliances that make things quicker and easier. In the light of this trend, air fryers are definitely a worthwhile kitchen appliance to invest in. They make it easier to cook the foods you adore and are a huge help whilst on a low-carb or keto diet. In addition to that, they make cooking at home more convenient and allow you to explore diverse cooking choices.

I hope you enjoyed this book and it has gotten your creative juices flowing. I trust it will help you shake up a tedious diet routine by giving you delightful and healthy meal ideas using an air fryer.

Remember, healthy eating doesn't have to be complicated, and you don't have to starve yourself to lose weight.

All there is left for me to say is: "Happy frying"!

Part 2

Is cooking with a deep fryer healthy?

Deep fryers are a healthy, guiltless way to enjoy your favourite fried food, that have become increasingly popular lately.

They are designed to help reduce the fat content of popular foods like fries, chicken wings, empanadas and fish fingers.

What is a fryer and how does it work?

A fryer is a popular kitchen appliance that cooks fried foods such as meat, pastries and potato chips.

It circulates hot air containing fine oil droplets around the food to create a crunchy and crispy appearance and taste.

This also results in a chemical reaction known as the Maillard effect which occurs in the presence of heat between an amino acid and a reducing sugar. This leads to changes in colour and taste of the food.

Air fried foods are a healthy alternative to fried foods thanks to their low-fat content and low caloric content.

Instead of dipping the food completely in the oil, you only need a tablespoon of oil for frying, to give the fried food a similar taste and a similar consistency.

Using an air fryer can help to reduce fat.

Deep-fried foods are generally more fatty than foods made using other cooking methods.

For example, a chicken breast that has been fried contains about 30% more fat than the same amount of roasted chicken.

Some manufacturers claim that using a fryer can reduce the fat content of fried foods by 75%.

In fact, fryers require much less fat than traditional fryers. While many fried dishes require up to 3 cups (750 ml) of oil, air fryers only need 1 tablespoon (15 ml).

This means that deep fryers consume up to 50 times more oil than fryers, and even if the oil is not completely absorbed by food, using an air fryer can significantly reduce fat content from your food.

A study compared the properties of deep-fried French fries and air fried French fries which showed that air frying resulted in a much lower fat end product with similar colour and moisture content.

This can have a significant impact on your health, as higher intake of vegetable oil fats has been linked to an increased risk of diseases such as heart disease and inflammation.

SUMMARY - Air fryers uses less oil than fryers and can produce foods with significantly lower fat content.

Moving to an air fryer can help you lose weight.

Air fried foods are not only lower in fat, but also lower in calories and can contribute to weight loss.

A study of 33,542 Spanish adults showed that increased consumption of fried foods was associated with an increased risk of obesity.

If you want to cut your waistline, you can start by replacing your fried foods with air fried foods.

With 9 calories in every gram of fat, fats contain twice as many calories per gram as other macronutrients like proteins and carbohydrates.

Because air fried foods are less fatty than fried foods, switching to an air fryer can be an easy way to reduce calories and promote weight loss.

SUMMARY – Air fried Foods are less fatty than fried foods that can help reduce calorie intake and promote weight loss.

Compared to frying, using an air fryer can reduce the amount of fat, calories, and potentially harmful compounds in your food.
However, air-fried foods are still fried foods and their regular consumption can be associated with health problems.

Although fryers may be a better alternative to deep fryers, limiting your consumption of fried foods is the best option for your health.

What are the benefits of air frying?

I am sure you have seen the excitement (online) with fryers! These devices are undoubtedly the most popular and trendy thing of cooking this year. Maybe you are curious what the hype is about?
The first time I heard about it, I was also curious. Why are people so excited about these things? How can frying be healthy?

These devices are not fryers. They look more like a small independent convection oven. They use electrical elements to quickly heat the air, and then circulate that hot air around and through your food. This hot air cooks the food fast, making the food golden and crispy, but the inside stays moist and delicious.

Advantages of cooking with a deep fryer

There are many reasons to use a fryer.

1. Cook healthier

So, how can frying be healthy? Easy! These units can be used without oil or with a small oil jet.

You can cook fries, onion rings, wings and more while getting really crisp results without extra oil. Compared to using my oven, the fries in the fryer were crisper but not dried out, and their use to cook breaded zucchini was even more impressive!

2. Faster meals

Since they are smaller than an oven and circulate the air around with fans, they cook food faster. An oven may take 20 to 30 minutes to heat properly, these fryers reach the temperature in minutes.

I was very impressed with the fact that my frozen fries were perfect after 15 minutes while they were in the oven for up to 45 minutes. If you need to make snacks or meals in a hurry, you will save time.

3. Versatility

I think that's my favourite feature of an air fryer. You can do so much with it! Yes, it fries very well compared to an oven. But it can also bake (even cake), broil, roast, grill and stir fry! Do you want chicken and peas for dinner? Easy to cook them with one of these.

You can prepare fresh and frozen food and even reheat leftovers. I made meat, fish, pans, sandwiches and many different vegetables in mine. Some fryers have additional features, like a rotisserie rack, grill pan or elevated cooking rack. With the divisible baskets you can cook several things at once. It is impressive to see that a unit can cook so many things in so many ways.

Depending on the size of your fryer you can buy many accessories. Cake and pizza pans, kebab skewers and steamer are just some of the accessories I've seen.

4. Space saver

If you have a small kitchen or live in a dorm or shared apartment, you can appreciate this benefit. Most of these units are about the size of a coffee machine. They do not take up too much space on the counter and are generally easy to store or move.

I appreciate the fact that they can replace other appliances like a toaster, and some people use them in kitchens in place of ovens.

5. Ease of use

Most fryers are very easy to use. Just choose the temperature and cooking time, add food and shake several times during cooking.

With the baskets you can shake your food easily and quickly and the device does not lose much heat when opened. So do not hesitate to check out if you want! Unlike an oven, you will not slow things down when you do it.

6. Easy cleaning

Part of the cooking that most of us do not appreciate is the cleaning. With an air fryer, you only have one basket and one pan to clean, and you can also use dishwasher. With non-stick coated parts, food does not normally stick to the pan. It only takes a few minutes to wash after use. It inspires me to cook more often at home, because I'm not afraid to clean!

7. Energy efficiency

These fryers are more efficient than using an oven. I used mine during a heat wave and I love that my kitchen is not hot when I use it. If you're trying to keep your home cool in the summer or worry about your electricity bills, you'll be impressed with the efficiency of these devices.

Who can benefit most from cooking with a fryer?

Everyone can benefit from using an air fryer, but this is especially good for some groups.

Busy parents

Need a quick snack after school? Late, but the kids ask for dinner? Just throw chips and nuggets in one of these dishes and prepare dinner in about 15 minutes! Parents love the speed with which they prepare food and the ease with which they have to clean up. It takes less time than getting a pizza!

Seniors

This is a great option for seniors who just do not want to keep a hot stove or prepare many ingredients. You can use frozen meat, pre-cut vegetables and seasonal dishes to your liking. They are so easy to use and will not tire your hands and can do anything from snacks to a full meal. Easy to clean.

Students

The ultimate snack! If it's one o'clock in the morning and you're writing an article, just throw wings or chips or make a grilled sandwich. With a deep fryer, you can become the most popular person in your dorm. Do not worry about the time that mess hall will close.

Easy

It can be difficult to be motivated to cook when living alone. It's just not worth heating the oven or spending a lot of time cutting things just to eat something. With a fryer you can prepare a small amount of food for a single serving in just a few minutes. Eat healthier and save money by not eating all the time! A deep-fryer is much more useful than a microwave and allows a lot of tasty food.

People who hate cooking

This is the ideal device for those who do not like to cook. You do not have to waste time, preparing ingredients for your food. You can use it with frozen meats like chicken wings, rib eye steaks and even frozen pizza. Make fries, onion rings, potatoes and nuggets in a few minutes. You can take a pack of pre-cut vegetables and make a quick stir fry. Grilled cheese sandwich sounds good? Go for it. Easy to use and clean, this fryer will not make you hate the kitchen.

Should I consider a fryer?

If you are fascinated by the benefits I mentioned, consider air frying. Perfect for small kitchens, dorms and offices, they enable you to prepare healthy meals quickly and easily. There are units of all sizes, from singles to large families, and they usually cost between $ 60 and $ 400. You can find the perfect device for your needs and cook the same evening.

How to preheat Air fryer?
A step-by-step guide and a few things to keep in mind:

1. Check the manual

The very first thing to do with any kind of electronic product is to read the manual. This also applies to a fryer. That way, you know exactly how to use the device, so you do not make mistakes or damage it.

This is very important for preheating, as some manufacturers may have their own preferred methods for this task. It is best to follow the instructions of these companies so that you do not cancel your warranty just because you want to use your new device.

2. Check the air fryer for cleanliness

Now that you know whether the manufacturer of your Air fryer has specific pre-heating instructions or not, the next step is to check the cleanliness of your device.

You need to be careful, as food remnants and debris can affect the taste of the next dish that you will prepare in the deep fryer.

The basket must be thoroughly cleaned and properly dried before use. Check every angle of your cooking basket to make sure nothing is left.

3. Connect the device

As an electrical appliance, your deep fryer must be connected in order to be used. Be careful, because not all fryers are equipped with a dual power supply.

If you are using a fryer that has been purchased in another country in the United States, check the voltage used by your location. The 120V appliances are grilled in a 220V outlet and deep fry the electrical components of your deep fryer, and nobody wants them. Always make sure first before connecting anything.

4. Put the accessories in place

If you want to use an accessory for your fryer, it is best to put it in the appliance before preheating. Therefore, the accessories can also be prepared for cooking. It will also make things easier if you do this step now.

If the fryer is already hot, you might not have ample grasp on it to place accessories securely. It is advisable to prepare the device at this point so that you do not have any problems later.

5. Turn on the device

The next step is pretty obvious: turn on your deep fryer. Without the unit that is ready and willing to go, no magic will be performed. Once you have read the manual, you need to know where the power switch is located. Just tap it and you're ready to preheat.

6. Set the timer

Now, when the device is on, you can preheat it. The next step would be to set the timer. Experts say preheating should take more than three minutes. Preheating is generally recommended for 5 minutes, although it may depend on the unit you own.

Some units with pre-heating instructions have their own note for the preheating time of the fryers. Refer to this information and you will not go wrong.

7. Select the highest temperature settings

Although the duration may vary from device to device, the temperature settings are completely different. Almost all manufacturers will tell you that you must set the appliance to the highest heat setting for preheating.

It may seem exaggerated, but in reality, it works very well. This will allow your fryer to reach the desired temperature in minutes, so follow this step.
When the timer has expired, you have finished preheating. You can now load the food and start cooking.

8. Don't have time? Add 3 minutes to your cooking time instead

As mentioned above, some fryers do not require preheating. You can do that as well, but with most prescriptions based on pre-heating times, this can discourage your cooking time.

To compensate for this, you can add 3 minutes to the timer setting for your recipe. In this way your ingredients are always cooked thoroughly and evenly.

If you think you do not want to preheat your fryer, you should also be prepared to make estimates and experiment.

You may need to check the doneness of your food several times before you reach the beautiful golden brown desired. A little patience may also be necessary if you ignore the preheating.

Final judgment

Even if you've never tried to work with an oven before, you do not have to worry about preheating your fryer.

The latter is a very basic cooking appliance, so you can be sure that preheating is not too difficult. You just have to know exactly what to do to get the job done.

Learning how to preheat the fryer takes just a few minutes of your time. However, it can bring fried, crispy and crunchy foods for a lifetime, so it's definitely worth it.

RECIPES

Avocado fries

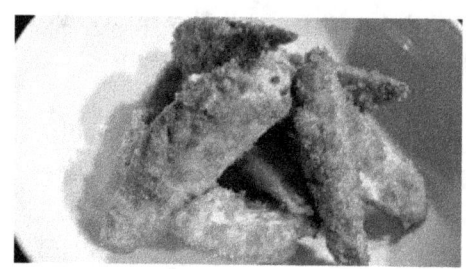

Active time
15 minutes
Total time
30 minutes
Yield
For 4 people (serving: 4 avocado pommes, 2 tablespoons sauce)

Avocado fries? Oh yeah! This irresistible combination of crispy and creamy is the ultimate treat of the air fryer. They are a bit heavier in calories than most of our snacks, but they are so good they are worth the occasional splurge!

The secret of the perfect air fryer, roasted avocado, is to choose avocados which are just ripe, but with sufficient strength to hold their shape while cooking. Paired with this spicy-hot sauce, these fries are excellent.

Ingredients

- 1/2 cup all-purpose flour
- 1 1/2 teaspoons of black pepper
- 2 eggs
- 1 tablespoon of water
- 1/2 cup panko (Japanese breadcrumbs)
- 2 avocados, each divided into 8 slices
- cooking spray
- 1/4 teaspoon kosher salt
- 1/4 cup ketchup without added salt
- 2 tablespoons of canola mayonnaise
- 1 tablespoon of apple cider vinegar
- 1 tablespoon chilli sauce

How to make avocados fries

1. Mix the flour and pepper in a bowl.

2. Beat eggs and water gently in a second bowl.

3. Put the panko in a third bowl.

4. Sprinkle the avocado in the flour.

5. Immerse the egg mixture and allow excess water to drip off.

6. Dredge in Panko, press to stick.

7. Coat avocado wedges well with cooking spray.

9. Place the avocado wedges in the air fryer and cook at 400 ° F until
golden, 7 to 8 minutes, turning avocado half way.

10. Remove from the air fryer; sprinkle with salt.

11. While the avocado are cooking stir ketchup, mayonnaise, vinegar and sriracha in a small bowl.

12. To serve, add 4 avocado fries to each plate with 2 tablespoons of sauce.

Roasted salmon with fennel salad

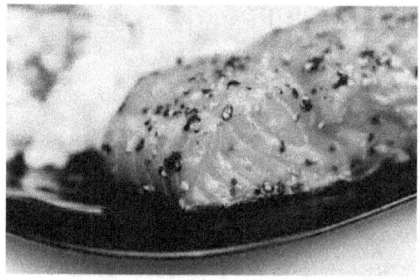

Your fryer has more up its sleeve than the crunchy stuff expected - it's also a fantastic oven for roasting meaty fish fillets like salmon. This recipe serves four, but you can easily cut it down by half to prepare a dinner for two.

Everything fits so well together - while the salmon is cooking, whip up the quick and tangy fennel slaw. When done, the salmon will be hot and ready to serve. For a little more heft, serve this meal with a side of your favourite fast-cooking brown rice.

Ingredients

- 2 teaspoons of finely chopped parsley

- 1 teaspoon finely chopped fresh thyme

- 1 teaspoon salt

- 4 salmon fillets cut in the middle without skin (6 oz)

- 2 tablespoons olive oil

- 4 cups chopped fennel (2 [15oz] fennel)

- 2/3 cup of Greek yogurt 2% fat

- 1 crushed garlic clove

- 2 tablespoons fresh orange juice (of 1 orange)

- 1 teaspoon of fresh lemon juice (of 1 lemon)

- 2 tablespoons chopped fresh dill

How to cook roasted salmon with fennel salad.

1. Preheat the oven to 200 ° F.

2. Mix the parsley, thyme and 1/2 teaspoon salt in a small bowl.

3. Brush the salmon with oil; sprinkle with the herb mixture.

4. Put 2 salmon fillets in the air fryer basket and cook at 350 ° F to the desired doneness, 10 minutes.

5. Transfer to the preheated oven to keep warm.

6. Repeat the process with the remaining fillets.

7. While the salmon is cooking, mix the fennel, yogurt, garlic, orange juice, lemon juice, dill, and the remaining 1/2 teaspoon of salt in a medium bowl.

8. Serve the salmon fillets over fennel salad.\

Southern-Style Chicken

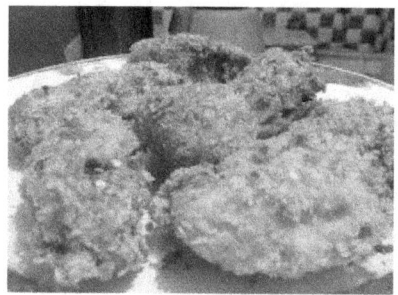

Ingredients

- 2 cups crushed Ritz Cracker (about 50)

- 1 tablespoon of chopped fresh parsley

- 1 teaspoon of garlic salt

- 1 teaspoon of paprika

- 1/2 teaspoon pepper

- 1/4 teaspoon ground cumin

- ¼ teaspoon sage

- 1 big beaten egg

- 1 broiler/fryer chicken (3 to 4 pounds), cut up

How to cook Southern-Style Chicken

1. Preheat the fryer to 375 °. Sprinkle the frying basket with a cooking spray.

2. Mix the first seven ingredients in a shallow bowl.

3. Place the egg in a separate shallow bowl.

4. Dip the chicken into the egg and then into the cracker mixture, tapping to stick the coating.

5. Put a few pieces of chicken in a single layer in the prepared basket, spray with cooking spray.

6. Bake for 10 minutes.

7. Turn chicken and spray with cooking spray; cook until the chicken is golden yellow and the juice is clear, 10 to 20 minutes longer.

8. Repeat with the rest of the chicken.

Air fried vegetables

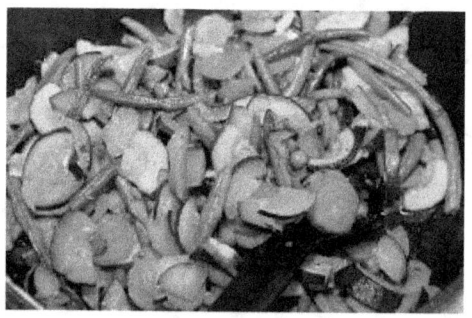

Use an air fryer to cook vegetables with perfectly delicate interiors and wonderfully crisp exterior.
Preparation time: 10 min
Cooking time: 20 min
Total time: 30 min
Servings: 4

Ingredients

- 1 pound / 0.5 kg vegetables (broccoli, Brussels sprouts, carrots, cauliflower, parsnips, potatoes, sweet potatoes, zucchini, etc.), evenly chopped

- 1 tablespoon / 30 ml cooking oil

- Salt and pepper

How to cook air fried vegetables

1. Preheat the air dryer for about 5 minutes at 182 ° C.

2. Chop the vegetables and mix with oil and salt and pepper. If you are preparing potatoes or sweet potato fries, soak them in water for about 30 minutes to extract the excess starch for crisp results, and then dry them thoroughly with paper towels.

3. Place the vegetables in the deep fryer and fry for 15 to 20 minutes, stirring the vegetables every 5 to 8 minutes.

4. Some vegetables need more time and others need less - use your judgment when opening the tray to stir vegetables.

5. You want the exterior to be golden and crisp and the interior to be delicate.

Air-Fried Ham & Egg Toast Cups

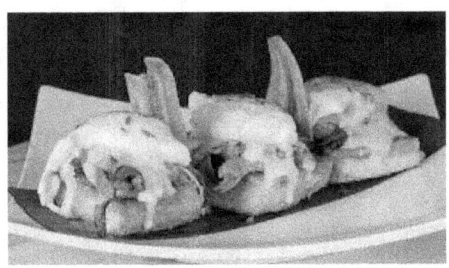

Ingredients:

- 4 Ramekins
- 4 eggs
- 8 slices of toast
- 2 slices of ham
- Butter
- Salt
- Pepper
- cheese (optional)

How to make Air-Fried Ham & Egg Toast Cups

1. First, brush the inside of the ramekin with a generous amount of butter with a baking brush. Seriously, the more butter, the easier it is to remove the cups of bread from the ramekins.

2. Flatten 8 slices of bread with a rolling pin or your own palm. Make it as flat as possible

3. Align the inside of each ramekin with a slice of toast. I know it's a bit strange to squash a square in a circle, and there's certainly an excess of bread that bends inward. But try to pinch the extra folds and make a cup as nice as possible.

4. Place another slice of flattened toast on top of the first toast and try to flatten the extra folds.

5. Cut 2 slices of ham into 8 smaller strips.

6. Place in each ramekin 2 pieces of ham.

7. Crack an egg into each toast cup.

8. Add a pinch of salt and ground black pepper to each egg

9. You can also add cheese to the toast cup. Personally, I use 1 slice of cheddar cheese and cut it into small pieces.

10. Place the 4 ramekins in the air fryer for 15 minutes at 160 degrees. You do not have to pre-heat the air fryer in advance

11. When finished, remove the ramekins from the air fryer with a cloth, silicone tweezers or other contraceptive methods to protect your fingers from heat.

12. To remove the toast cup from the ramekins, use a small knife and cut it slowly around the inside of the ramekin in case bread was stuck to the sides. Then turn the cup of ramekin toast with the same knife and a spoon.

Air fryer pickle

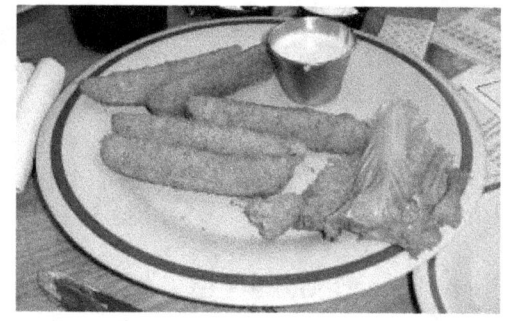

A pickle a day keeps the doctor away.

Proceeds: 4 servings

TIME OF PREPARATION: 0 HOUR 10 MIN

TOTAL TIME: 0 HOURS 20 MIN

Ingredients

2 cup dill pickle slices

1 egg, beaten with 1 tablespoon of water

3/4 cup breadcrumbs

1/4 cup freshly grated Parmesan cheese

1 tablespoon dried oregano

1 tablespoon garlic powder

Ranch, to serve

How to make Air fryer pickle

1. Dry the pickle with paper towels.

2. In a medium bowl mix breadcrumbs, parmesan, oregano and garlic powder.

3. Dredge pickle chips first in egg and then in the breadcrumb mixture.

4. Place in a fryer and cook for 10 minutes at the highest temperature.

5. Serve immediately, with ranch for soaking.

Parmesan chicken

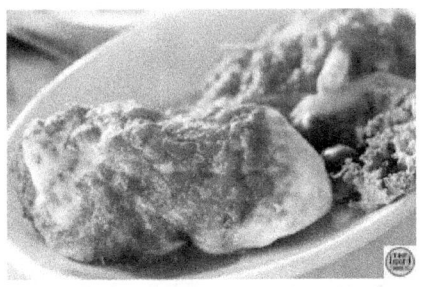

4 points freestyle 251 calories

TOTAL TIME: 30 minutes

The Parmesan chicken is great in the fryer, you do not have to use so much oil!

Ingredients:

- Cut 2 chicken breasts (about 8 oz) in half to form 4 slices
- 6 tablespoons of spiced breadcrumbs
- 2 tablespoons of grated Parmesan
- 1 tablespoon of melted butter (or olive oil)
- 6 tablespoon light mozzarella
- 1/2 cup of marinara
- cooking spray

How to make parmesan chicken

1. Preheat the fryer at 360 ° f for 9 minutes.
2. Spray the basked lightly.
3. Combine the breadcrumbs and Parmesan in a bowl.
4. Melt the butter in another bowl.
5. Lightly brush the butter on the chicken and dip it into the breadcrumb mixture.

6. When the fryer is ready, put 2 pieces in the basket and sprinkle with oil at the top.

7. Bake for 6 minutes, turn over and garnish with 1 tablespoon of sauce and 1 1/2 tablespoons of grated mozzarella.

8. Bake for 3 minutes or until the cheese has melted.

9. Set aside and keep warm, repeat with the other 2 pieces.

Manchurian Gobi

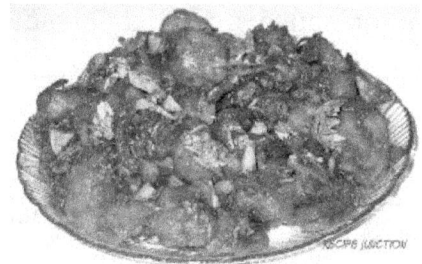

Ingredients

For the sauce

- 1 tablespoon canola oil
- 2 tablespoon chopped garlic
- 2 tablespoon chopped ginger
- 1 small red onion diced
- 3 chopped scallions
- 2/3 cup vegetable broth, plus a little more if needed
- 1/3 cup sambal

For the batter

- 1/2 cup of AP flour
- Corn starch 1/2 cup, plus 1-4 Tablespoon extra

- 2 teaspoon Onion powder
- 2 teaspoon of garlic powder
- 1 teaspoon garam masala
- 1 teaspoon of salt
- 1/2 teaspoon black pepper
- 1/2 teaspoon turmeric
- 1/2 cup of water

For cauliflower

- 1 small cauliflower head cut into small pieces
- canola, grapeseed or vegetable oil, for frying
- 2 servings of basmati rice prepared
- chopped cilantro for garnish

How to make Manchurian Gobi

Sauce

1. Heat the oil in a medium saucepan over medium heat. Add garlic and ginger and sauté until soft, but not browned (about 7 minutes).

2. Add the red onions and scallions and mix. Add liquid to the pan as needed to soften the vegetables but not turn brown (10-15 minutes).

3. At this point, the vegetables should be soft and most of the liquid absorbed. Remove from heat and stir in the desired amount of sambal. Put aside.

Batter

1. Combine all batter ingredients in a medium bowl, except corn-starch and water.

2. Add water, stir gently and add one extra corn starch with one tablespoon after the other to get a smooth consistency. You want it to be thin enough to cover the cauliflower florets, but not too thin that it drips too fast or too thick that it doesn't cover florets evenly.

Cauliflower

1. Put the florets in a large pot. Cover with water and put a lid on it. Bring to a boil, than remove from heat and drain. Transfer them to a baking tray with a refrigerated shelf to allow the cauliflower to cool.

2. Add a few inches of oil to a small cast iron pot or deep fryer and heat to 325-350 degrees.

3. Add several florets to the batter and carefully add one after the other to the hot oil. Fry till golden, then transfer to paper towels with a skimmer to drain, as you repeat the process with the rest of the florets. Do not overload the pot or your florets will stick together.

4. Mix the fried florets into the prepared sauce, then place in an air fryer at 400 degrees for 8 to 10 minutes and shake them every few minutes to avoid sticking. (Depending on the size of your air fryer, you may need to do this in 2 to 4 batches.)

5. Serve immediately with prepared basmati rice and chopped cilantro.

Air Fryer Churros With Chocolate Sauce

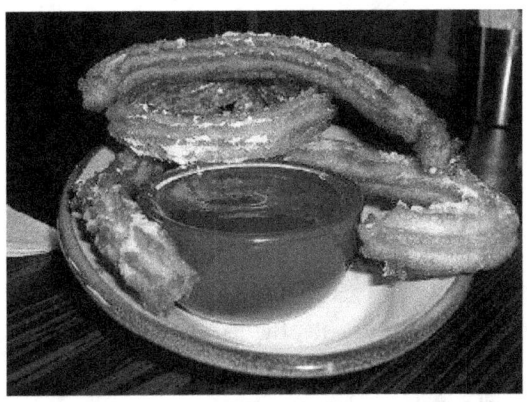

These delicacies are lighter than traditional churros - almost like éclairs - and come out of the fryer and are mild and delicious. The mixture of cinnamon and sugar forms a thin crust on the outside, which allows to preserve this classic crunch.

Kefir is a dairy product similar to yogurt, which is much thinner (it's drinkable, like a smoothie) and contains healthy probiotics. The slightly sour taste makes the chocolate sauce pleasant and supple. Be sure to cool the dough before channelling it in the frying basket.

You will enjoy the churros immediately because they are fresh, but you can keep any extra chocolate sauce.

Ingredients

- 1/2 cup of water
- 1/4 teaspoon salt
- 1/4 cup, plus 2 tbsp. unsalted butter
- 1/2 cup flour
- 2 big eggs
- 1/3 cup of granulated sugar
- 2 teaspoons of ground cinnamon
- 4 ounces of sweet chocolate finely chopped
- 3 tablespoons heavy cream
- 2 tablespoons of vanilla kefir

How to cook churros with chocolate sauce

1. Add water, salt and 1/4 cup butter in a small saucepan over medium heat to a boil.

2. Reduce the heat to medium-low; Add the flour and stir vigorously with a wooden spoon until the dough is smooth, about 30 seconds. Continue cooking until the dough comes off the sides of the pan and a film forms at the bottom of the pan, 2 to 3 minutes.

3. Put the dough in a medium bowl.

4. Stir constantly until slightly cooled, about 1 minute.

5. Add the eggs, 1 at a time, stirring constantly until they are completely smooth after each addition.

6. Transfer the mixture to a piping bag with a middle star tip. Cool 30 minutes.

7. Pipe 6 (3 inches long) pieces in a single layer in the basket of an air fryer. Bake at 380 ° F until golden, about 10 minutes.

8. Repeat with the remaining dough.

9. Mix sugar and cinnamon in a medium bowl. Brush churros with the remaining 2 tablespoons of melted butter and roll them into the sugar mixture to coat.

10 Put the chocolate and cream in a small microwave-proof bowl.

11. Microwave until the mixture is melted and smooth, about 30 seconds, stirring after 15 seconds.

12. Stir in the kefir. Serve the churros with a chocolate sauce.

Spicy roasted chicken breasts

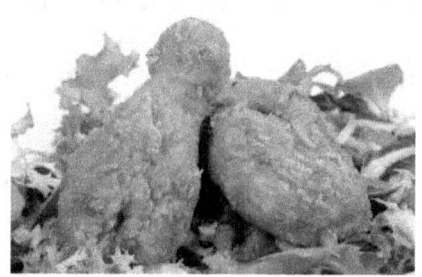

Ingredients

- 2 cups of buttermilk

- 2 tablespoons of Dijon mustard

- 2 teaspoons of salt

- 2 teaspoons of hot pepper sauce

- 1 teaspoons of garlic powder

- 8 bone in chicken breasts, without skin (8 ounces each)

- 2 cups of soft breadcrumbs

- 1 cup cornmeal

- 2 tablespoons of canola oil

- 1/2 teaspoon poultry seasoning

- 1/2 teaspoon ground mustard

- 1/2 teaspoon paprika
- 1/2 teaspoon cayenne pepper
- 1/4 teaspoon dried oregano
- 1/4 teaspoon dried parsley flakes

How to make Spicy roasted chicken breasts

1. Preheat the fryer to 375 °.

2. In a large bowl, combine the first five ingredients.

3. Add chicken and turn to coat. Refrigerate, covered, 1 hour or overnight.

4. Drain the chicken, discarding marinade. Mix the remaining ingredients in a shallow bowl and stir to combine.

5. Add the chicken, piece by piece and turn to coat.

6. Place in an air fryer basket with cooking spray in a single layer.

7. Fry in the air fryer until a thermometer indicates 170 °, turning halfway, about 20 minutes.

8. Repeat with the rest of the chicken.

9. When the last serving of chicken is cooked, put the whole chicken back in the basket and air fry it for 2 to 3 minutes to heat.

Spanish frittata with potatoes and chorizo

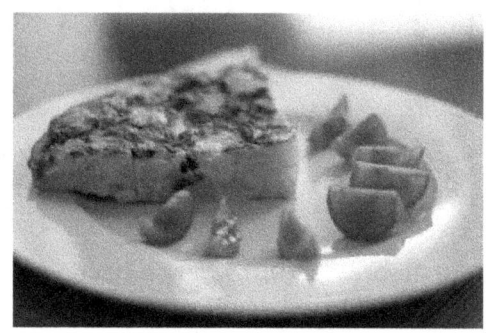

Ingredients

3 eggs

½ Chorizo sausage

1 large potato - cooked and diced

½ cup of frozen corn

olive oil

parsley

½ wheel of feta

salt and pepper

How to make Spanish frittata with potatoes and chorizo

1. Pour a good amount of olive oil into the pan of the air fryer (or your pan on stove) and add the chorizo, corn and potatoes.

2. Set the fryer to 180 ° C and cook the sausages and potatoes until lightly browned.

3. Break the 3 eggs in a small bowl and beat with a fork.

4. Season with salt and pepper.

5. Put the eggs with the potato and the sausage in the pan and garnish with chopped feta and parsley.

6. Cook another 5 minutes, check and cook for another minute if necessary.

7. At the end of cooking, put on a plate and serve with a tasty tomato sauce and a fresh rocket.

8. If you do it on the stove and oven, preheat the oven to 180 ° C and cook the potato and sausage in a baking pan.

9. When the potato is lightly browned, beat the eggs in a small bowl and pour over the potato and sausage.

10. Garnish with feta cheese and parsley and bake until the eggs are cooked.

Bourbon bacon burgers

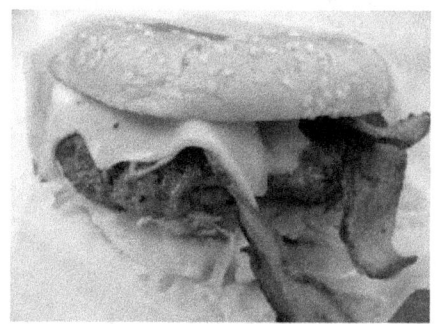

Ingredients

- 1 tablespoon of bourbon

- 2 tablespoons of brown sugar

- 3 pieces of maple bacon halved

- ¾ lbs beef

- 1 tablespoon of chopped onion

- 2 tablespoons barbecue sauce

- ½ teaspoon salt

- freshly ground black pepper

- 2 slices of Colby Jack cheese (or Jack Monterey)

- 2 Kaiser rolls

- Tomato and lettuce for serving

Zesty Burger Sauce:

- 2 tablespoons barbecue sauce

- 2 tablespoons mayonnaise

- ¼ teaspoon ground paprika

- freshly ground black pepper

How to make Bourbon bacon burgers

1. Preheat the fryer to 390ºF and pour some water into the bottom of the fryer. (This prevents the grease that drops in the bottom drawer from burning and smoking.)

2. Mix bourbon and brown sugar in a small bowl. Put the bacon strips in the air fryer basket and brush with the brown sugar mix.

3. Air fry at 400 ° F for 4 minutes. Turn the bacon over, sprinkle with brown sugar and air fry for another 4 minutes at 390ºF until crispy.

4. While the bacon is cooking, prepare the burger patties.

5. In a large bowl, mix ground beef, onion, barbecue sauce, salt and pepper.

6. Gently mix with your hands and shape the meat into 2 patties.

7. Place the hamburger patties in the air fryer basket and fry the burgers at 370 ° F for 15 to 20 minutes, depending on how you like your burger (15 minutes for rare to medium food).

8. While the burgers are air frying, prepare the burger sauce by combining the BBQ sauce, mayonnaise, paprika, and freshly ground black pepper to taste in a bowl.

9. When the burgers are cooked to your taste, top up patty with a slice of Colby Jack cheese and air fry for another minute just to melt the cheese. (You can attach the cheese slice to the burger with a toothpick to prevent it from being blown into the fryer.)

10. Put the sauce inside the Kaiser rolls, place the burgers on the rolls and garnish with the bacon, salad and tomatoes and enjoy!

Smoky sweet crunchy chickpeas

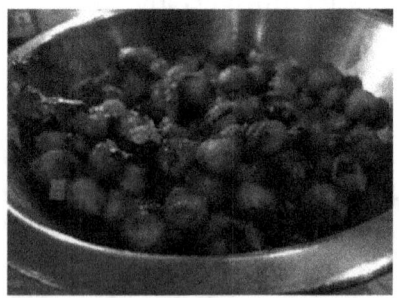

Ingredients:

1 (15 ounces) can chickpeas

2 tablespoons of chickpea aquafaba

1 tablespoon of maple syrup

2 teaspoons of smoked paprika

1 1/2 teaspoons of garlic powder

1/2 teaspoon sea salt

How to cook sweet crunchy chickpeas

1. Drain the chickpeas by reserving Aquafaba. Do not rinse the chickpeas.

2. Put the chickpeas into the air fryer, shake in a layer and place inside the fryer. Fry at 400 ° F for 8 minutes.

3. While cooking the chickpeas: In a bowl, whisk 2 tablespoons of aquafaba, maple syrup, smoked paprika, garlic powder and salt. (Save the rest of the Aquafaba for another use.)

4. Add fresh chickpeas from air fryer and stir to coat. Return the flavored chickpeas to the frying basket with a spatula to get all the sauce.

5. Put the chickpeas back into the air fryer. Fry at 390 ° F for another 5 minutes. Shake the basket and return to the fryer for 3 to 5 minutes until the chickpeas are crispy.

6. Put in a serving bowl. Serve warm or at room temperature - as an aperitif, salad or snack!

Strawberry tart

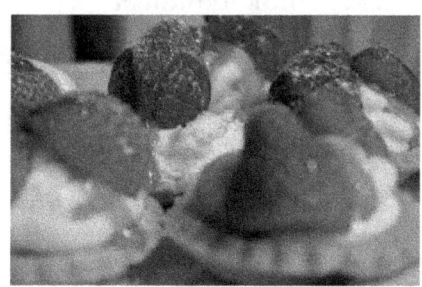

Ingredients

8 oz. Halved strawberries (about 1 3/4 cups)

1/4 cup sugar

(14.1 oz.) PKG pieces

cooking spray

1/2 cup (about 2 ounces) caster sugar

1 1/2 teaspoon fresh lemon juice (1 Lemon)

1/2 oz sweets arc-en-ciel (about 1 tbsp.)

How to make strawberry tart

1. Mix strawberries and granulated sugar in a microwave safe bowl.

2. Let it rest for 15 minutes, stirring occasionally.

3. Microwave at high heat, until shiny and reduced, about 10 minutes, stirring during halfway of cooking.

4. Cool completely for about 30 minutes.

5. Roll the pie crust into a 12-inch circle on a lightly floured surface.

6. Cut the dough into 12 rectangles (2 1/2 x 3 inches) and roll the pieces again if necessary.

7. Pour about 2 teaspoons of strawberry mixture into the middle of 6 rectangles of dough, leaving a 1/2 inch border.

8. Brush the edges of the dough rectangles with water; top with remaining dough rectangles, then press the edges with the fork to seal.

9. Coat the tarts with a cooking spray.

10. Place 3 tarts in a single layer in a frying basket and bake at 350 ° F until golden brown, about 10 minutes. Repeat with the remaining tarts. Place on a wire rack to cool completely, about 30 minutes.

11. Mix sugar and lemon juice in a small bowl until smooth.

12. Spoon glaze over cooled tarts and sprinkle evenly with candy.

Air Fryer Garlic-Rosemary Brussels Sprouts

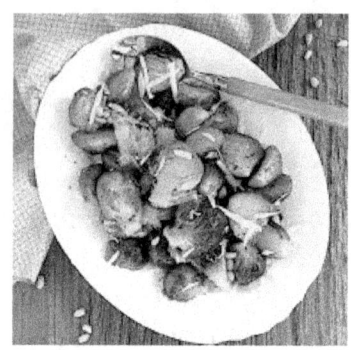

Ingredients

- 3 tablespoons of olive oil
- 2 garlic cloves chopped
- 1/2 teaspoon salt
- 1/4 teaspoon pepper
- 1 lb. Brussels sprouts trimmed and cut in half
- 1/2 cup panko breadcrumbs (Japanese)
- 1 teaspoons of freshly chopped rosemary

How to cook Air Fryer Garlic-Rosemary Brussels Sprouts

1. Preheat the air fryer to 350 °. Put the first four ingredients in a small microwave-safe bowl; Microwave on high for 30 seconds.

2. Mix Brussels sprouts with 2 tablespoons of oil mixture.

3. Put all Brussels sprouts in air frying basket and cook for 4-5 minutes.

4. Continue air frying, stirring every 4 to 5 minutes, until the sprouts are almost tender and lightly browned, for about 8 minutes.

5. Mix breadcrumbs with rosemary and remaining oil mixture; sprinkle the sprouts. Continue cooking until the crumbs are golden and the sprouts are tender, 3 to 5 minutes. Serve immediately.

Smoked pork chops with raspberry

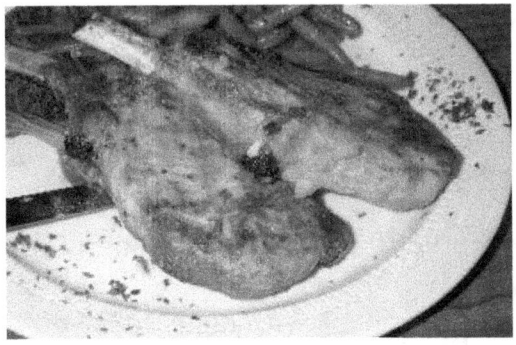

Ingredients

- 2 large eggs

- 1/4 cup of milk
- 1 cup Panko breadcrumbs (Japanese)
- 1 cup of finely chopped pecans
- 4 pork chops, smoked (7-1 / 2 ounces each)
- 1/4 cup all-purpose flour
- 1/3 cup balsamic vinegar
- 2 tablespoons of brown sugar
- 2 tablespoons of raspberry jam without seeds
- 1 tbsp of frozen orange juice

How to make Smoked pork chops with raspberry

1. Preheat the fryer to 400 °.
2. Spray fryer with cooking spray.
3. Whisk eggs and milk in a shallow bowl.
4. In another flat bowl, mix breadcrumbs with pecans.
5. Coat pork chops with flour; shake off the surplus.
6. Dip into the egg mixture, then into the crumb mixture, patting to help in sticking.

7. Work in batches as needed, place chops in a single layer in the basket of the air fryer; spray with a cooking spray.

8. Cook until golden yellow for 12 to 15 minutes turning halfway through cooking and spray with another cooking spray.

9. Remove and keep warm.

10. Repeat with the remaining chops.

11. In the meantime, put the remaining ingredients in a small saucepan; bring to a boil.

12. Cook and stir until thickened, 6-8 minutes. Serve with chops.

Breakfast style air fryer potato

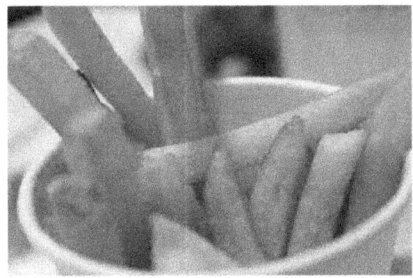

Ingredients

2 medium potatoes (cut into about 1-inch pieces)

• oil spray

• pinch of salt and pepper

• 1 small pepper (~ 5 ounces or about 3/4 cup), medium hard

• 1 small onion (~ 4 ounces or about 3/4 cup), chopped medium

How to make Breakfast style air fryer potato

1. Put the potatoes in the basket of the fryer.

2. Spray with oil, shake, spray again and add a pinch of salt.

3. Set the air fryer to 400 degrees for ten minutes. Stop once to shake during the cooking time. (Do not hesitate to move if the potatoes are not moving enough)

4. After the potatoes have cooked for 10 minutes, add the peppers and onions.

5. Add another spray of oil and shake the basket. Set the air fryer to 400 degrees and cook for 15 minutes.

6. Check during the last 5 minutes that the potatoes are not too brown.

7. Depending on the size of your potatoes, you may need a little less time or a little more time.

8. If necessary, add a few extra minutes to the cooking time.

9. Add salt to taste and serve.

Cinnamon rolls

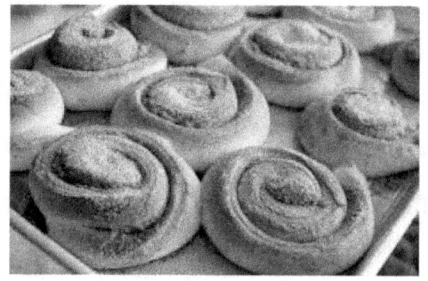

Ingredients

- 1 pound of frozen bread dough, thawed
- ¼ cup melted and cooled butter
- ¾ cup brown sugar
- 1 ½ tablespoons of ground cinnamon

Cream cheese glaze:

- 4 ounces of cream cheese, softer
- 2 tablespoons soft butter
- 1¼ cup powdered sugar
- ½ teaspoon of vanilla

How to make Cinnamon rolls

1. Let the bread dough on the counter come to room temperature. On a lightly floured surface, roll the dough into a 13 "x 11" rectangle. Place the rectangle with the 13-inch side facing you. Spread the melted butter over the whole dough, leaving a 1-inch edge along the edge furthest away from you.

2. Mix the brown sugar and cinnamon in a small bowl. Sprinkle the mixture evenly over the buttered dough and keep the edge of 1 inch uncovered. Roll the dough in a log starting at the edge closest to you. Roll the dough tight, making sure you roll evenly. When you reach the open edge of the dough, squeeze the dough to seal it.

3. Cut the log into 8 pieces and cut it slowly with a sawing motion so as not to flatten the dough. Turn the slices on the sides and cover them with a clean cloth. Let the rolls rest for 1 ½ to 2 hours in the hottest corner of your kitchen.

4. For the glaze, place the cream cheese and butter in a microwave-safe bowl. Soften the mixture for 30 seconds in the microwave until it is easy to stir.

5. Gradually add the powdered sugar and mix. Add the vanilla extract and stir until smooth. Put aside.

6. When the rolls are raised, preheat the fryer to 350ºF.
Put 4 rolls in the basket of the deep fryer. Air fry for 5 minutes. Turn the rolls over and let them jump for another 4 minutes. Repeat with the other 4 rolls.

7. Allow the rollers to cool for a few minutes before glazing. Spread large spoons of cream cheese over the cinnamon rolls and allow some glaze to flow on the side of the roll. Serve hot and enjoy!

Easy falafel recipe (GLUTEN FREE)

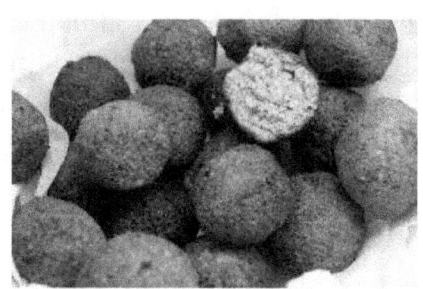

Ingredients

- 16 oz of dried chickpeas
- 1 small yellow onion sliced
- 2 cloves of garlic
- 1/2 bunch of chopped fresh parsley
- 1/4 bunch of chopped fresh cilantro
- 1 tablespoon of cumin
- 1/4 tsp. cayenne pepper
- black pepper, to taste
- 1 1/2 tsp. Salt tea
- 1/2 lemon juice

- 1/4 cup chickpea flour *
- 2 tablespoons of Tahini

How to cook Easy falafel recipe (GLUTEN FREE)

1. Preheat your air fryer to 350 F.

2. Put soaked chickpeas, chopped onion and garlic in a large food processor.

3. Process until the mixture finely chopped but not mush.

4. Then add the fresh herbs, dried spices and lemon juice. Repeat until the mixture is well incorporated - the mixture should turn green.

5. Finally, add the chickpea flour and tahini to the food processor and process until well combined.

6. Transfer the falafel mixture into a large bowl and use your hands to form round balls with about 2 tablespoons of mixture.

7. In the air fryer: bake for 18 minutes at 350 ° F, turn over and cook for another 15 to 18 minutes.

8. Put 1 tablespoon of heat-sensitive oil in the pan for 5 falafel balls.

9. Fry over medium heat and turn the balls about every 2 minutes to brown all sides. This process takes about 20 minutes.

10. Serve as desired. Falafel dries easily in the fridge but keeps well in a sealed container for up to 5 days.

Doughnut

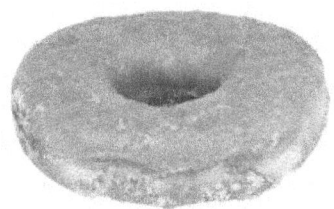

If you crave donuts, these fermented rings offer the same sweet, delicate and crispy sweetness with your air fryer.

Ingredients

- 1/4 cup of warm water

- 1 teaspoon of active dry yeast

- 1/4 cup plus 1/2 teaspoon. granulated sugar divided

- 2 cups of all-purpose flour

- 1/4 teaspoon kosher salt

- 1/4 cup whole milk, at room temperature

- 2 tablespoons unsalted butter melted

- 1 big beaten egg

- 1 cup (4 ounces) powdered sugar

- 4 teaspoons of tap water

How to make doughnuts

1. Mix the water, the yeast and 1/2 teaspoon of granulated sugar in a small bowl; Let stand for about 5 minutes.

2. Mix the flour, salt and the remaining ¼ cup of granulated sugar in a medium bowl.

3. Add the yeast mixture, milk, butter and egg; Mix with a wooden spoon to make soft dough.

4. Turn the dough over a lightly floured surface and knead for 1 to 2 minutes. Put the dough in a lightly greased bowl.

5. Cover and allow to rise in a warm place until the volume is doubled, about 1 hour.

6. Turn the dough on a lightly floured surface. Gently roll to 1/4 inch thick.

7. Cut 8 donuts with a 3-inch circular cutter and a 1-inch circular cutter to remove the centre. Place doughnuts on a lightly floured surface.

8. Cover with plastic wrap and let rest for about 30 minutes until doubling.

9. Place 2 donuts and 2 donut holes in a single layer in the air fryer basket and bake at 350 ° F until golden, 4 to 5 minutes. Repeat with the other donuts.

10. Whisk the powdered sugar and water in a medium bowl until smooth. Dip donuts and donut holes in the glaze.

11. Place on a baking sheet on a baking tray so that excess glaze glass can drip off. Let stand until the glaze hardens, about 10 minutes.

Air Fryer coconut shrimp and Apricot Sauce

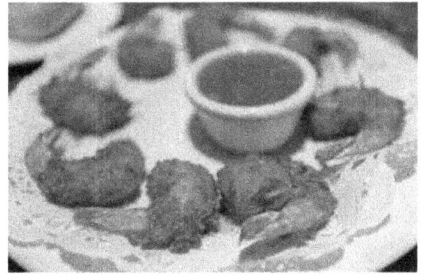

Ingredients

- 1/2 pound raw raw shrimp

- 1-1 / 2 cup sweet coconut flakes

- 1/2 cup panko breadcrumbs (Japanese)

- 4 egg whites

- Hot sauce in Louisiana

- 1/4 teaspoon salt

- 1/4 teaspoon pepper

- 1/2 cup all-purpose flour

Sauce:

- 1 cup of apricot preserves

- 1 teaspoon apple cider vinegar

1/4 teaspoon minced red pepper flakes

How to cook Air Fryer coconut shrimp and Apricot Sauce

1. Preheat the fryer to 375 °.

2. Peel and remove the shrimp leaving the tails.

3. In a shallow bowl, mix the coconut with the breadcrumbs.

4. In another flat bowl whisk egg whites, spicy sauce, salt and pepper.

5. Put the flour in a third bowl.

6. Dip the prawns in the flour to coat well; shake off the surplus. Dip into the egg white mixture, then tap into the coconut mixture to adhere the coating.

7. Spray the grease basket with a cooking spray. When working in batches as needed, place the shrimp in a single basket in the air fryer.

8. Cook for 4 minutes; turn shrimp and cook until the coconut is lightly browned, about 4 minutes.

9. In the meantime, place the ingredients of the sauce in a small saucepan; Cook and stir over medium heat until canned. Serve the shrimp immediately with the sauce.

Hash brown

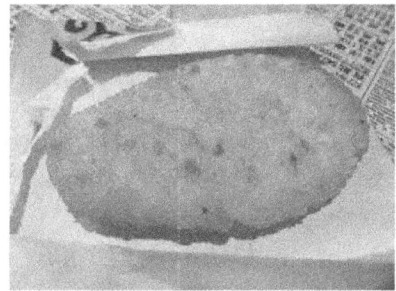

This hash brown recipe is almost oil free, you can use a little oil for this fryer recipe.

Ingredients

- Large potatoes - 4 - peeled and finely grated

- corn flour - 2 tablespoons

- salt - to taste

- Pepper powder - to taste

- Chilli flakes - 2 teaspoons

- garlic powder - 1 teaspoon

- onion powder - 1 teaspoon

- Vegetable oil - 1 + 1 teaspoon

How to cook hash brown

1. Soak the grated potatoes in cold water. Empty the water. Repeat the step to drain the excess starch from the potatoes.

2. In a non-stick pan, heat 1 teaspoon of vegetable oil and fry the grated potatoes until lightly cooked for 3 to 4 minutes.

3. Cool the potatoes and place on a plate.

4. Add the cornmeal, salt, pepper, garlic and onion powder and chili flakes and mix well.

5. Distribute on the plate and tap firmly with your fingers.

6. Refrigerate it for 20 minutes.

7. Preheat the fryer to 180 ° C.

8. Take out the now cooled potato and divide it into equal pieces with a knife.

9. Brush the wire basket of the fryer with a little oil.

10. Put the browned potato pieces in the basket and fry at 180 ° C for 15 minutes.

11. Take out the basket and flip the hash browns at 6 minutes to make it evenly fried.

12. Serve hot with ketchup.

Nashville hot chicken

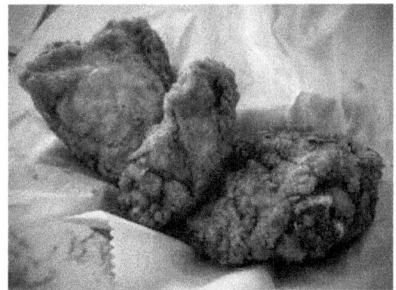

Ingredients

- 1 chicken (4 pounds), cut into 6 pieces (2 breasts, 2 thighs and 2 drumsticks)

- 2 eggs

- 1 cup buttermilk

- 2 cups of all-purpose flour

- 2 tablespoons of paprika

- 1 teaspoon of garlic powder
- 1 teaspoon of onion powder
- 2 teaspoons of salt
- 1 teaspoon of freshly ground black pepper
- vegetable oil

Nashville Hot Sauce

- 1 tablespoon of cayenne pepper

- 1 teaspoon of salt

- ¼ cup of vegetable oil

- 4 slices of white bread

- Dill pickle slices

How to cook Nashville hot chicken

1. Cut the chicken breast into 2 pieces, so you have a total of 8 pieces of chicken.

2. Install a two-stage dredging station. Whisk eggs and buttermilk in a bowl.

3. Mix the flour, paprika, garlic powder, onion powder, salt and black pepper in a lockable plastic zippered bag.

4. Dip the chicken pieces into the egg-buttermilk mixture and pour into the seasoned flour on all sides.

5. Repeat this process (egg mixture and flour mixture) again. This can be a bit complicated, but make sure that all sides of the chicken are completely covered.

6. Spray the chicken with vegetable oil and set aside.

7. Preheat the fryer to 370ºF. Spray or brush the bottom of the basket with a small vegetable oil.

8. Fry the chicken twice at 370 ° F for 20 minutes and turn the pieces after cooking. Transfer the chicken to a plate, but do not cover it.

9. Repeat with the second batch of chicken.

10. Lower the temperature of the fryer to 340 ° F. turn the chicken and place the first batch of chicken on the second batch that is already in the basket.

11. Air fry for 7 minutes.

12. While the chicken is frying, mix cayenne pepper and salt in a bowl.

13. Heat the vegetable oil in a small pot and when it is very hot, add it to the spice mixture and stir it smooth.

14. It sizzles briefly when you add it to the spices.

15. Put the fried chicken on top of white bread and brush the hot sauce over the chicken.

16. Top with pickle slices and serve hot. Enjoy the warmth and the taste!

Spicy kale chips

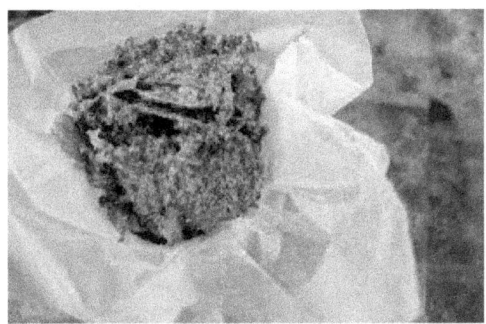

These slightly crunchy, spicy kale fries are the perfect salty snack.

Ingredients

- 1 large bunch of kale, destemmed, washed and spun - torn into bite-sized pieces (about 3 cups)

- 1 tablespoon of olive oil

- 1 to 2 tablespoons Za'atar spice

- ½ - 1 teaspoon sea salt

How to cook spicy kale chips

1. Put your washed and dried kale in a large bowl and mix the olive oil.

2. Gently massage the olive oil into the kale with your hands until it is well covered.

3. Add the spices and mix well

4. Place the kale in portions in the basket of your air fryer, set at 170 ° C.

5. The chips should be ready when the edges are brown but not burnt.

6. Be sure to have eye (and nose) on them while cooking.

5. If you do not have a fryer, you can bake it on a parchment-lined baking tray at 170 degrees in your oven. It should take about 10-15 minutes in a preheated oven.

Lighten up Empanadas in an Air Fryer

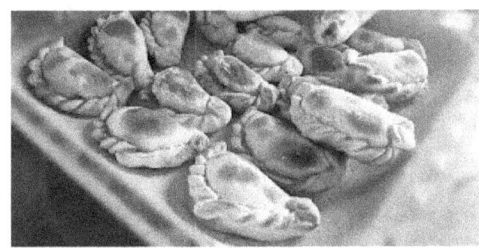

Ingredients

- 1 tablespoon of olive oil

- 3 oz (85/15) lean ground beef

- 1/4 cup finely chopped white onion

- 3 ounces of finely chopped Cremini mushrooms

- 2 teaspoons of finely chopped garlic

- 6 green olives, pitted, chopped

- 1/4 teaspoon paprika

- 1/4 teaspoon ground cumin

- 1/8 teaspoon of ground cinnamon

- 1/2 cup chopped tomatoes

- 8 square gyoza wrappers

- 1 big egg slightly beaten

How to make Lighten up Empanadas in an Air Fryer

1. Heat the oil in a medium sized pan at medium heat.

2. Add beef and onion; cook, stir to crumble until it starts to brown, 3 minutes.

3. Add the mushrooms and stir occasionally until the mushrooms begin to turn brown, 6 minutes.

4. Add garlic, olives, paprika, cumin and cinnamon; cook until the mushrooms are very tender and they have liberated most of their liquid, 3 minutes.

5. Stir in the tomatoes and cook for 1 minute with occasional stirring.

6. Put the filling in a bowl and let it cool for 5 minutes.

7. Arrange 4 gyoza wrappers on the work surface.

8. Place about 1 1/2 tablespoons of filling in the middle of each pack.

9. Coat the edges of the packaging with eggs; Fold the wrappers and press the edges to seal them.

10. Repeat the process with the remaining wrappers and fillings.

11. Place 4 empanadas in a single layer in a frying basket and bake at 400 ° F until golden brown, 7 minutes.

12. Repeat this with the other empanadas.

Air Fryer Bourbon Bacon Cinnamon Rolls

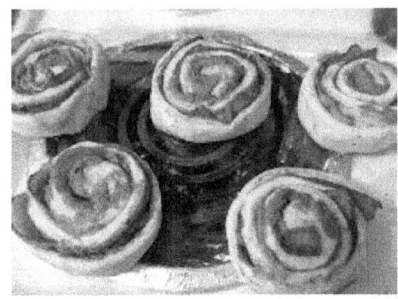

Ingredients

- 8 bacon strips

- Bourbon 3/4 cup

- 1 tube (12.4 ounces) of chilled cinnamon rolls with icing

- 1/2 cup of chopped pecans

- 2 tablespoons of maple syrup

- 1 teaspoon chopped fresh ginger

How to cook Air Fryer Bourbon Bacon Cinnamon Rolls

1. Put the bacon in a bowl; Add bourbon.

2. Seal and cool it for the whole night. Next day Remove the bacon and pat dry; Throw the bourbon.

3. In a large pan, cook the bacon in batches over medium heat until almost crispy, but still soft.

4. Remove to paper towels to drain.

5. Dispose of all juices except a teaspoon.

6. Preheat the air fryer to 350 °. Separate the dough into eight rolls by reserving icing packet.

7. Unwind the spiral rollers in long strips; pat the dough to 6x1-inches strips.

8. Place a strip of bacon on each strip of dough and cut bacon as needed; Charming, forming a spiral. Pinch the ends to seal.

9. Repeat with the remaining dough. Transfer four rolls into the basket of the air fryer; cook 5 minutes.

10. Turn the rolls over and cook until golden, about 4 minutes.

11. In the meantime, mix pecans and maple syrup. Mix the ginger in another bowl with the contents of the ice packet.

12. In the same pan, heat the remaining bacon juice over medium heat. Add the pecan mixture; cook, stirring frequently, until lightly browned, 2-3 minutes.

13. Sprinkle half of the glaze on hot cinnamon rolls; Cover with half of the pecans. Repeat the process to create a second batch.

Air fryer French Toast Sticks Recipe

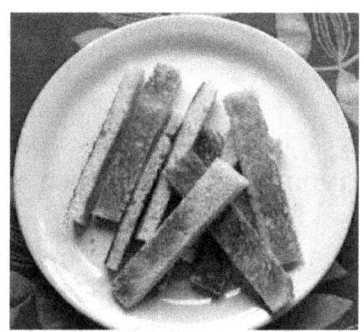

Ingredients

- 4 pieces of sliced bread

- 2 tablespoons butter or margarine

- Beat 2 eggs gently

- Salt

- cinnamon

- nutmeg

- ground clove

- Powdered sugar and / or maple syrup for garnishing and serving

How to cook Air fryer French Toast Sticks Recipe

1. Preheat air fryer to 180 * Celsius.

2. Beat two eggs in a bowl, a pinch of salt, a few cinnamon and a pinch of nutmeg and cloves.

3. Butter both sides of the slices of bread and cut into strips.

4. Put each strip into the egg mixture and arrange it in the air fryer (you must cook in two batches)

5. Stop the air fryer after 2 minutes of cooking time, remove the pan, make sure the pan is placed on a heat-resistant surface, and spray the bread with a cooking spray.

6. Once you have generously coated the strips, turn them over and spray the second side as well

7. Put the pan back in the fryer and cook for another 4 minutes. After a few minutes, check that they cook evenly and that they do not burn.

8. When the egg is cooked and the bread is golden brown, remove it from the air fryer and serve it immediately.

9. For garnishing and serving, sprinkle with powdered sugar,
sprinkle with whipped cream, drizzle with maple syrup or serve with a small bowl of syrup.

Air Fryer Jalapeno Poppers

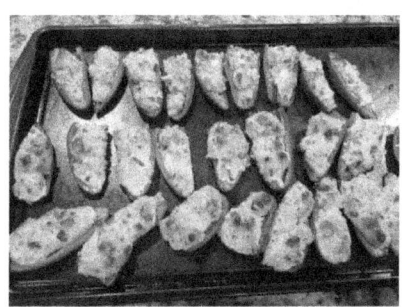

Ingredients

- 10 jalapeno peppers halved
- 8 ounces of cream cheese
- 1/4 cup fresh parsley
- Gluten -free tortilla 3/4 c or breadcrumbs

How to cook Jalapeno Poppers

1. Mix half of the crumbs and cream cheese together. Once combined, add the parsley.

2. Fill each pepper with this mixture.

3. Gently squeeze the top of the peppers into the remaining 1/4 c crumbs to create the top layer.

4. Cook in air fryer at 370 degrees F for 6 to 8 minutes or in a conventional oven at 375 degrees F for 20 minutes.

5. Let cool and enjoy!

Peach pies

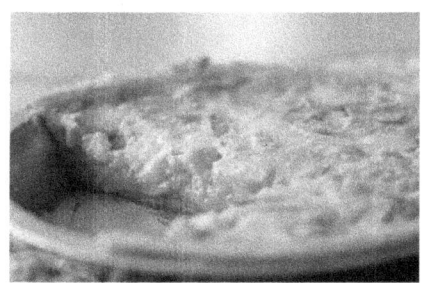

Ingredients

- 2 fresh peaches (5 ounces), peeled and chopped
- 1 tablespoon of fresh lemon juice (of 1 lemon)
- 3 tablespoons of sugar
- 1 teaspoon of vanilla extract
- 1/4 teaspoon of table salt
- 1 teaspoon corn-starch
- 1 pkg (14.1 oz) pie crust
- cooking spray

How to make peach pies

1. Mix peaches, lemon juice, sugar, vanilla and salt in a medium bowl.

2. Let rest for 15 minutes and stir occasionally. Drain peaches, reserving 1 tablespoon of liquid.

3. Stir corn starch into the reserved liquid; stir into drained peaches.

4. Cut the piecrust into 8 (4-inch circles).

5. Put about 1 tablespoon of stuffing in the middle of each circle.

6. Coat the edges of the dough with water.

7. Fold the dough over the filling to form half-moon.

8. Crimp the edges with a fork to seal; Cut 3 small slits into the top of the pies.

9. Cover the pies well with a cooking spray.

10. Place 3 pies in a single layer in the frying basket and bake at 350 ° F until golden, 12 to 14 minutes.

Air Fryer Chocolate Chip Oatmeal Cookies

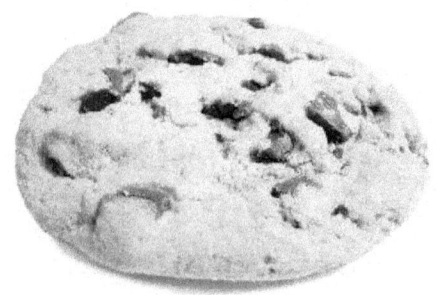

Ingredients

- 1 cup of soft butter
- 3/4 cup of sugar
- 3/4 cup brown sugar
- 2 big eggs
- 1 teaspoon of vanilla extract
- 3 cups of instant cooking oats
- 1-1 / 2 cup all-purpose flour
- 1 pack (3.4 ounces) vanilla pudding mix
- 1 teaspoon baking soda
- 1 teaspoon of salt
- 2 cups (12 ounces) of semi-sweet pieces of chocolate chips
- 1 cup of chopped nuts

How to cook Chocolate Chip Oatmeal Cookies

1. Preheat the air fryer to 350 °.

2. Line the basket of the fryer with aluminium foil.

3. In a large bowl, stir cream butter and sugar. Beat eggs and vanilla.

4. Mix oatmeal, flour, dried pudding mix, baking soda and salt;

5. Gradually add to the cream mixture and mix well.

6. Stir in chocolate chips and nuts.

7. Form balls with a tablespoon of dough; flatten easily.

8. Place the dough 2 inches apart on the fryer basket.

9. Air fry for 8-10 minutes or until lightly browned.

10. Remove to wire rack. Repeat with the remaining dough.

Airfryer beetroot chips

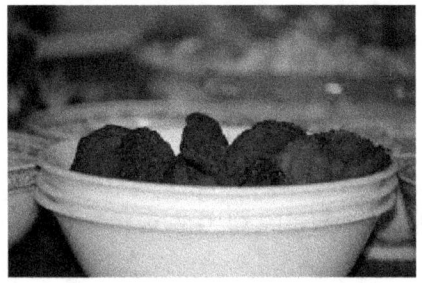

Even if you hate beetroot, try it !! You will love these beet chips.

Ingredients

- 2 medium-sized beetroot

- 1/2 teaspoon of oil

- salt to taste

- Pepper optional

How to cook beetroot chips

1. Wash beetroot, peel and remove skin.

2. Cut into thin slices with a mandolin cutter.

3. Otherwise, if you do not have a cutting machine, cut it evenly with your knife.

4. Use the skin to dye your accessories if you wish or dispose of them in your food waste.

5. Divide the beet slices onto the paper and place another piece of paper on top.

6. Keep it aside for 10 minutes. This process absorbs extra moisture on the turnips.

7. Sprinkle the necessary salt on the beets.

8. Preheat the Air fryer to 150 ° C for 4 minutes.

9. Remove the basket from the air fryer and put the chips in it.

10. Slide it into the air fryer and fry for 15 minutes.

11. Be sure to remove and shake well every 5 minutes.

12. Once the fries are crispy on the outside edges and tender in the middle, let them cool for a while.

13. Slide the basket with the chips and heat for another 3 minutes at 180 ° C. The chips will be sharp and perfect.

14. If necessary, season with sea salt and freshly ground pepper or just snorkel on it.

Taco Bell crunch wraps

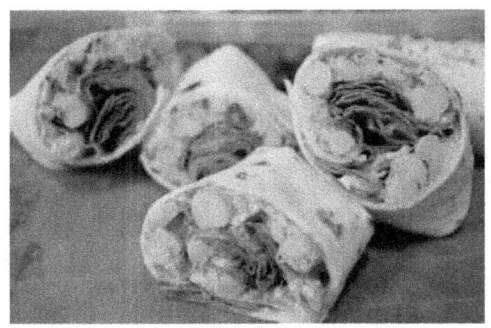

Ingredients

2 pounds of ground beef

2 sachets of taco seasoning

1 1/3 cup of water

6 flour tortillas 12 inches

3 tomatoes Roma

12 ounces nacho cheese

2 cups shredded salad

2 cups Mexican cheese

2 cups sour cream

6 Tostadas

Olive oil or butter spray

How to cook Taco Bell crunch wraps

1. Preheat the fryer to 400.

2. Prepare meat according to tacos seasoning manual.

3. Fill the middle of each tortilla with 2/3 c beef, 4 tablespoons Nacho cheese, 1 Tostada, 1/3 c sour cream, 1/3 c salad. 1/6 c of tomatoes and 1/3 c of cheese

4. To close, flood the edges up, over the middle, this should look like a pinwheel.

5. Repeat 2 and 3 with the remaining wraps.

6. Put the curved side in your fryer.

7. Spray with oil.

8. Cook for 2 minutes or until brown.

9. Carefully turn over with a spatula and spray.

10. Cook another 2 minutes and repeat with the other wraps.

Homemade Croutons

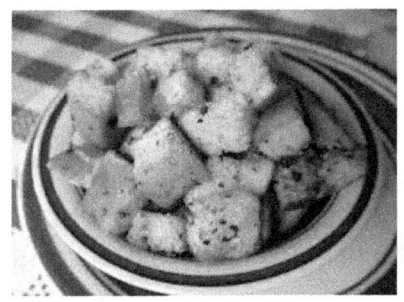

Ingredients

6 slices
First batch

3-4 tablespoon spreadable butter

Dried parsley

Batch two

2 tablespoons olive oil

Dried parsley

Sprinkle with pepper

garlic powder

How to make homemade croutons

1. Place 3 slices of bread on top of each other and cut into cubes.

2. Cut them a bit bigger because the slices of bread shrink a bit.

3. Having the edges or removing them is your personal choice. I retain them for my croutons.

4. Prepare a mixture of melted butter and dried parsley in a large bowl. Spread them on bread.

5. Preheat the Air fryer to 160 ° C for 3 minutes.

6. After heating, place the bread cubes in the tray and air fry them together for 7 to 8 minutes. At this time, the bread cubes on the outer surface are slightly crisp and very light brown in colour.

7. After 8 minutes, turn the dial in your air fryer to 180 ° C and air fry for 4 to 6 minutes.

8. The perfect golden croutons (bread cubes) are served with your salad or your tasty soup.

9. Repeat this process with your second batch.

Calzones

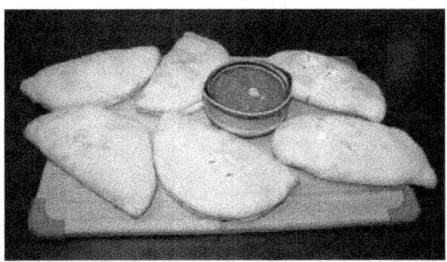

Ingredients

- 1 teaspoon of olive oil

- 1/4 cup finely chopped red onion (from 1 small onion)

- 3 ounces of spinach leaves (about 3 cups)

- 1/3 cup of sodium marinara sauce

- 2 ounces of grated chicken breast (about 1/3 cup)

- 6 ounces of freshly prepared whole wheat pizza dough

- 1 1/2 ounces pre-shredded mozzarella cheese (about 6 tablespoons)

- cooking spray

How to cook Calzones

1. Heat the oil in a medium to medium non-stick pan.

2. Add the onion and cook, stirring occasionally for 2 minutes.

3. Add the spinach; cover and cook until wilted for 1 1/2 minutes.

4. Remove the pan from the heat; stir marinara sauce and chicken.

5. Divide the dough into 4 equal pieces.

6. Roll each piece over a lightly floured surface in a 6-inch circle.

7. Add a quarter of the spinach mixture to half of each circle of dough.

8. Garnish each with a quarter of the cheese.

9. Fold the dough over the filling to form half-moons and squeeze the edges to seal them.

10. Coat the calzones well with a cooking spray.

11. Place the calzone in the frying basket and bake at 325 ° F until golden brown, after 8 minutes turn the calzone.

12. Cook total for 12-15 minutes.

Air fryer fish and fries

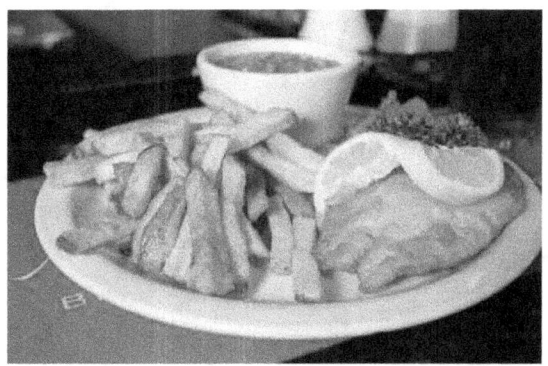

Ingredients

- 1 pound of potatoes (about 2 medium)

- 2 tablespoons olive oil

- 1/4 teaspoon pepper

- 1/4 teaspoon salt

FISH

- 1/3 cup all-purpose flour

- 1/4 teaspoon pepper

- 1 big egg

- 2 tablespoons of water

- 2/3 cup crushed cornflakes
- 1 tablespoon of grated Parmesan cheese
- 1/8 teaspoon cayenne pepper
- 1/4 teaspoon salt
- 1 pound of haddock or cod fillets
- tartar sauce, optional

How to cook air fryer fish and fries

1. Preheat the fryer to 400 °.

2. Peel and cut the potatoes lengthwise into 1/2-inch-thick slices; Cut the slices into 1/2 inches thick sticks.

3. Combine the potatoes in a large bowl with oil, pepper and salt. Put the potatoes in a single layer in an air fry basket; cook until tender, 5-10 minutes.

4. Mix the potatoes in the basket to redistribute; cook until lightly browned and crispy, 5 to 10 minutes longer.

5. Meanwhile mix flour and pepper in a bowl.

6. In another bowl, whisk the eggs with water.

7. In a third bowl mix cornflakes with cheese and cayenne pepper.

8. Sprinkle fish with salt; dip into flour mixture to coat both sides; shake off the surplus.

9. Dip into the egg mixture, then into the cornflake mixture, tapping to stick the coating.

10. Remove the chips from the basket; keep warm.

11. Put the fish in a frying basket in a single layer.

12. Cook until the fish is lightly browned and simply flake off with the fork.

13. Do not overcook.

14. Put the chips back in the basket to heat them.

15. Serve immediately, serve with tartar sauce.

Pork taquitos

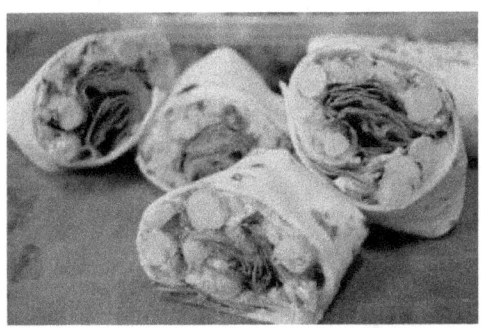

Ingredients:

Cooked 30 oz grated pork tenderloin (not a pork fan - use grated chicken instead!)

2 1/2 cups of grated mozzarella cheese

10 small tortillas

1 lime, juiced

cooking spray

Salsa for dipping

Sour cream

How to cook Pork taquitos

1. Preheat the fryer to 380 degrees.

2. Sprinkle lime juice over the pork and mix gently.

3. Microwave 5 tortillas at once with a damp paper towel for 10 seconds to soften.

4. Add 3 oz. of pork and 1/4 cup cheese to a tortilla.

5. Carefully roll the tortillas.

6. Put the tortillas on a pan covered with greased aluminium foil.

7. Apply a uniform layer of cooking spray on the tortillas.

8. Air fry for 7-10 minutes, until the tortillas have a golden colour, flipping hallway through.

Risotto balls

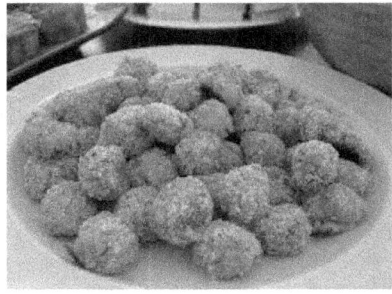

Ingredients

Risotto
- 1 tablespoon olive oil
- 1 cup of very small onion cubes
- 4 cups vegetable broth
- 1 cup Arborio rice
- 1 cup of Parmesan

loaf
- 1.5 cup breadcrumbs
- 2 beaten eggs

How to make Risotto balls

1. Add the olive oil to a large saucepan over medium heat.

2. Heat oil, add onions and sauté until soft.

3. Add the dry rice and fry for 1 minute.

4. Then add 2 cups of vegetable broth. Let the broth boil while stirring continuously to avoid burns.

5. Once the liquid has boiled, add another 2 cups. Continue this process until all of your fluid is absorbed and your rice are tender. This process should take about 20 minutes.

6. Add the risotto to a casserole or saucepan. Let it cool for 1 to 2 hours in the refrigerator. (This step is very important; the risotto must be cold to be rolled into balls).

7. Put the bread crumbs in a small bowl. In another bowl lay the beaten eggs.

8. Remove the chilled risotto (rice mixture) from the refrigerator.

9. Roll 1-inch rice balls. Dip it in the eggs and then into the breadcrumbs to coat the whole ball.

10. Do this until you run out of ingredients.

11. Place the rolled and coated balls in the refrigerator for 45 minutes.

12. Remove from the refrigerator and place in fryer in small quantities for frying.

13. Cook at 400 degrees F for a cooking time of 10 minutes.

14. The balls are actually around the 6-7 minutes, but tanning occurs only in the 8-10 minutes.
    13. Serve with Marinara Sauce and enjoy!

Fried chicken wings

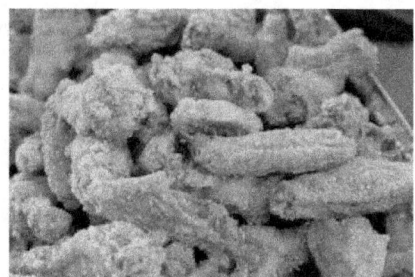

Ingredients

- 10 chicken drumettes (about 1 1/2 pounds).
- cooking spray.
- 1 tablespoon of low sodium soy sauce.
- 1/2 teaspoon corn starch.
- 2 teaspoons of honey
- 1 teaspoon of Sambal Oelek (ground fresh chili paste)
- 1 teaspoon finely chopped garlic
- 1/2 teaspoon finely chopped fresh ginger
- 1 teaspoon of fresh lime juice (from 1 lime)
- 1/8 teaspoon kosher salt
- 2 tablespoons of chopped shallots

How to cook fried chicken wings

1. Dry the chicken with paper towels. Coat chicken with cooking spray.

2. Place the chicken in the basket of the deep fryer, with percussion on the sides to avoid overfilling.

3. Bake at 400 ° F until the skin is very crispy, 25 minutes.

4. Whisk soy sauce and corn starch in a small pan.

5. Stir in honey, sambal, garlic, ginger, lime juice and salt.

6. Simmer over medium heat; simmer until the mixture begins to bubble and thicken.

7. Put the chicken in a bowl. Add the sauce and stir to coat well.

8. Sprinkle with green onions.

Green tomato BLT

Ingredients

- 2 medium green tomatoes (about 10 ounces)

- 1/2 teaspoon salt

- 1/4 teaspoon pepper

- 1 big beaten egg
- 1/4 cup all-purpose flour
- 1 cup Panko breadcrumbs (Japanese)
- 1/2 cup of mayonnaise
- 2 green onions finely chopped
- 1 teaspoon fresh dill or 1/4 teaspoon dill weed
- 8 slices of wholegrain bread toasted
- 8 bacon strips cut in the middle
- 4 Bibb or Boston lettuce leaves

How to cook Green tomato BLT

1. Preheat the deep fryer to 350 °.

2. Spray basket with cooking spray.

3. Cut the tomato into eight slices about 1/4 inch thick.

4. Sprinkle tomato slices with salt and pepper.

5. Put egg, flour and breadcrumbs in separate shallow bowls.

6. Dip the tomato slices in the flour, shake the excess, then dip into the egg and finally into the breadcrumb mixture, tapping to help stick properly.

7. Work in batches as required, place tomato slices in a frying basket in one layer; spray with a cooking spray.

8. Cook for 8 to 12 minutes until golden brown and spray with additional cooking spray.

9. Remove and keep warm; Repeat with the remaining tomato slices.

10. In the meantime, mix mayonnaise, spring onions and dill.

11. Spread each of the four slices of bread with two strips of bacon, a lettuce leaf and two slices of tomato.

12. Spread the mayonnaise mixture over the remaining slices of bread.

Healthy fish finger sandwich

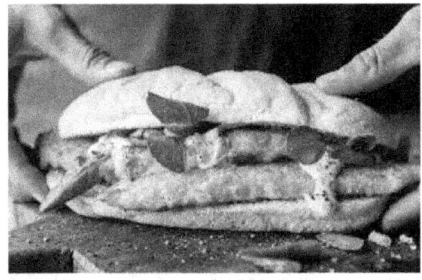

Ingredients

- 4 small cod fillets (skin removed)

- Salt and pepper
- 2 tablespoons of flour
- 40 g of dried breadcrumbs
- Spray oil
- 250 g frozen peas
- 1 tablespoon of fresh cream or Greek yogurt
- 10-12 capers
- squeeze out the lemon juice
- 4 bread rolls or 8 small slices of bread

How to cook healthy fish finger sandwich

1. Preheat the air fryer.

2. Take the cod fillets, season with salt and pepper and lightly sprinkle with flour.

3. Then quickly roll into the breadcrumbs.

4. The idea is to get a thin layer of breadcrumbs on the fish rather than a thick layer.

5. Repeat this with every cod fillet.

6. Put some oil sprays in the bottom of the frying basket.

7. Place cod fillets on top and cook for 15 minutes (200 C).

8. While the fish is cooking, boil the peas for a few minutes on the stove or in the microwave in boiling water.

9. Drain water and add to the blender with cream, capers and lemon juice. Blitz until combined.

10. Once the fish is cooked, remove it from the Air Fryer and start layering your sandwich with the bread, fish and peas. You can also add salad, tartar sauce and other favourite ingredients!

Fried bananas S'mores

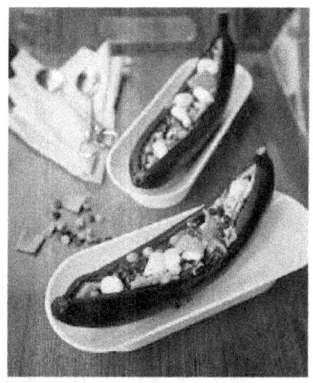

Ingredients

• 4 bananas.

• 3 tablespoons of semi-sweet chocolate chips

- 3 tablespoons of mini peanut butter chips

- 3 tablespoons of mini marshmallows

- 3 tablespoons cereal

How to make fried banana S'mores

1. Preheat the deep fryer to 400 ° F.

2. Cut the unpeeled bananas lengthwise on the inside of the curve, but do not cut them off at the bottom of the peel.

3. Open the banana lightly to form a pocket.

4. Fill each bag with chocolate chips, peanut butter chips and marshmallows.

5. Poke the graham cracker muesli into the filling.

6. Place the bananas in the frying basket and place them resting on each other to keep them upright with the filling.

7. Air fry for 6 minutes or until the banana feels soft, the skin is blackened, and the chocolate and marshmallows are melted and grilled.

8. Let it cool for a few minutes and then serve it with a spoon.

Curried Sweet Potato Oven Fries with Creamy Cumin Ketchup

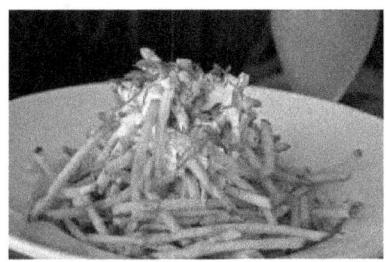

Ingredients

For sweet potato fries

- 2 sweet potatoes
- 2-3 tablespoons of olive oil
- 1/2 teaspoon curry powder
- 1/4 teaspoon coriander
- 1/4 teaspoon sea salt

For creamy ketchup with cumin

- 1/4 cup ketchup
- 2 tablespoons of mayonnaise
- 1/2 teaspoon ground cumin

- 1/8 teaspoon ground ginger

- a pinch of cinnamon

How to make Curried Sweet Potato Oven Fries with Creamy Cumin Ketchup

Make sweet potato fries

1. Preheat oven to 400F. (If you are baking, no fryer required.)

2. Cut your sweet potatoes in about 1/4? Sticks. They should be about as wide as your little finger, but longer is okay.

3. Place the sweet potato slices on a baking sheet and sprinkle with 2 tablespoons of olive oil.

4. Sprinkle with curry powder, coriander and sea salt.

5. Oven Instructions: Bake for 45 to 60 minutes, stirring every 15 minutes to cook evenly. When they look brown and a bit crunchy, they're done.

6. Instructions for the fryer: Transfer the sweet potato into the basket of your air fryer. Bake at 370F for 20 minutes with stirring after 10 minutes.

Make the Creamy Cumin Ketchup
Whisk all of the ingredients together in a small bowl.

Mexican corn in an air fryer

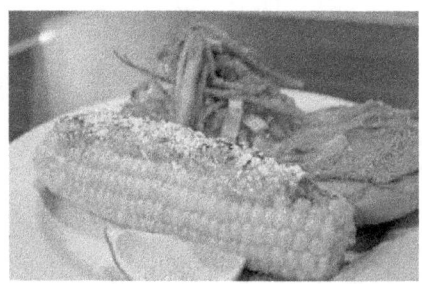

Ingredients

- 4 ears of fresh corn (about 1 1/2 lb.)

- cooking spray

- 1 tablespoon unsalted butter

- 2 teaspoons of chopped garlic

- 1 teaspoon of lime zest plus 1 tsp. fresh fruit juice (from 1 lime)

- 1/2 teaspoon kosher salt

- 1/2 teaspoon black pepper

- 2 tablespoons chopped fresh cilantro

How to make Mexican corn in an air fryer

1. Lightly cover the corn with a cooking spray and put it in a single layer in the air fryer basket.

2. Bake at 400 ° F until tender and lightly charred, 14 minutes, turning corn after half cooking.

3. In the meantime mix butter, garlic, lime zest and lime juice in a small microwave-safe bowl.

4. Microwave until butter melts, about 30 seconds.

5. Put the corn on a bowl and pour the butter mixture over it.

6. Sprinkle with salt, pepper and cilantro.

7. Serve immediately.

Lemon biscuits

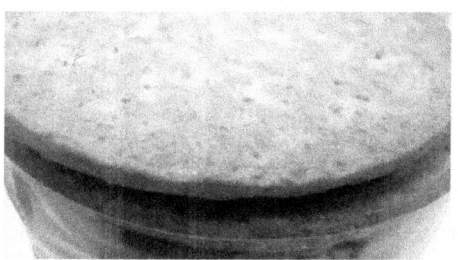

Ingredients

- 1/2 cup unsalted butter softened

- 1 pack (3.4 oz.) Instant Lemon Pudding Mix

- 1/2 cup of sugar

- 1 big egg

- 2 tablespoons milk 2%
- 1-1 / 2 cup all-purpose flour
- 1 teaspoon baking soda
- 1/4 teaspoon salt

Icing:

- 2/3 cup powdered sugar
- 2 to 4 teaspoons of lemon juice

How to make Lemon biscuits

1. In a large bowl, stir butter, pudding mix and sugar. Beat in egg and the milk.

2. Add flour, baking powder and salt in cream mixture and beat them properly.

3. Divide the dough in half. Form a 6 "inch long roll on a lightly floured surface, wrap and refrigerate for 3 hours.

4. Preheat the deep fryer to 325 °. Unwrap the dough and cut it crossways into 1/2 inches. Place the slices in a single layer in an air fryer basket.

5. Bake until the edges are light brown, 8-12 minutes.

6. Cool in the basket 2 minutes. Remove the cables to cool them completely. Repeat with the remaining dough.

7. Mix the sugar and lemon juice in a small bowl.

8. Drizzle on biscuits. Let it stand until it's done.

- Preparation: The dough can be prepared 2 days in advance. Wrap and place in a resealable container. Store in the fridge

- Freeze option: Place the packaged newspapers in a resealable container and freeze them. Unpack the frozen logs and slice them.

Cook as directed, increase the time by 1-2 minutes.

Air fried potato recipe - potatoes with parsley and garlic

Ingredients

3 potatoes

1-2 tablespoons olive oil

1 tablespoon salt

1 tablespoon of garlic

1 teaspoon of parsley

How to cook Air fryer baked potato

1. Wash your potatoes and make air holes with a fork in the potatoes.

2. Sprinkle with olive oil and spices, then rub the spices evenly over the potatoes.

3. Once the potatoes are coated, place them in the fryer basket and place them in the machine.

4. Air fry your potatoes at 392 degrees for 35 to 40 minutes or until tender.

5. Top up with your favourite topping. We like fresh parsley and sour cream!

Nutrition posts
    Air fried potato recipe - potatoes with parsley and garlic
    Quantity per serving
    Calories 213
    Total fat 4g
    Carbohydrates total 39g
    Protein 4g

Air fryer buffalo cauliflower

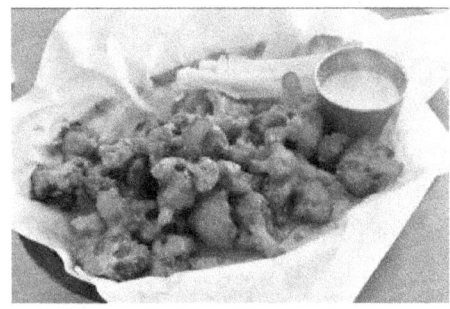

Ingredients

- 1 medium cauliflower, cut into 1 1/2 "florets (about 6 cups)

- 2-3 tablespoons Frank red hot sauce

- 1 1/2 teaspoon maple syrup

- 2 teaspoons of avocado oil

- 2-3 tablespoons of nutrient yeast (more for a cheese flavor, I use 3)

- 1/4 teaspoon sea salt

- 1 tablespoon corn starch

How to make Air fryer buffalo cauliflower

Instructions for air frying

1. Set the fryer to 360 degrees F.

2. Add all ingredients except cauliflower in a large mixing bowl.

3. Whisk to mix well.

4. Add cauliflower and mix to coat.

5. Add half of your cauliflower to the air fryer (no need to oil the basket).

6. Cook for 12 to 14 minutes, stirring while cooking or until the desired consistency is achieved.

7. Repeat with the remaining cauliflower, except lower cooking time to less than 9-10 minutes.

8. Cauliflower will be safe in the refrigerator for up to 4 days.

9. To warm up, place in the fryer for 1 to 2 minutes until it is warm and slightly crispy.

OVEN ROASTING INSTRUCTIONS

1. Preheat the oven to 415 degrees.

2. Lay out a baking tray with non-stick parchment paper.

3. Repeat the instructions for preparing the sauce and mix / coat the cauliflower. Spread the cauliflower evenly on a baking sheet.

4. Bake for 40 minutes, cook until the cauliflower has golden brown edges.

Make delicious whole wheat pizza in an air fryer

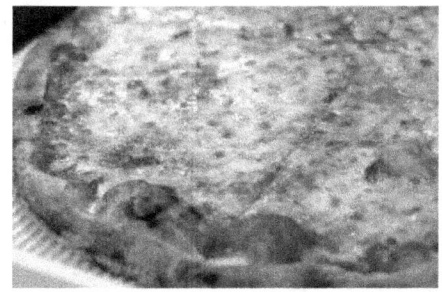

Ingredients

- 1/4 cup of sodium marinara sauce
- 2 whole wheat pita round
- 1 cup of spinach leaves (1 ounce)
- Cut 1 small tomato into 8 slices
- 1 small garlic clove chopped
- 1 oz partially sliced mozzarella cheese (about 1/4 cup)
- 1/4 oz Parmigiano-Reggiano cheese (about 1 tablespoon)

How to make whole wheat pizza in an air fryer

1. Distribute the marinara sauce evenly on one side of each pita bread.

2. Garnish with half the spinach leaves, sliced tomatoes, garlic and cheese.

3. Put 1 pita in the frying basket and bake at 350 ° F until the cheese melts and the pita is crispy, 4 to 5 minutes.

4. Repeat with the rest of the pita

Lava cakes with peppermint

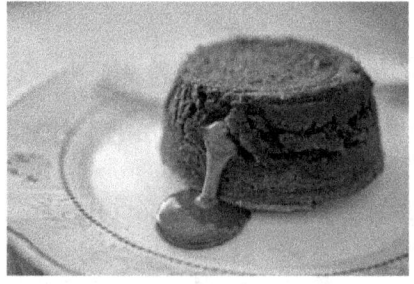

Ingredients

- 2/3 cup of semi-sweet pieces of chocolate
- 1/2 cup butter diced
- 1 cup icing sugar
- 2 big eggs
- 2 large egg yolks

- 1 teaspoon peppermint extract

- 6 tablespoons all-purpose flour

- 2 tablespoons finely ground mints, optional

How to cook lava cake with peppermint

1. Preheat the fryer to 375 °.

2. In a microwaveable bowl, melt the chocolate chips and butter for 30 seconds; stir until smooth.

3. Mix powdered sugar, eggs, egg yolks and extract until a smooth mixture is obtained.

4. Stir in the flour.

5. generously grease and flour four, 4-oz. ramekins; pour the dough into the ramekins.

6. Do not overfill. Put the ramekins in the air fryer basket; cook until a thermometer indicates 160 ° and the edges of the cakes are set, 10 to 12 minutes. Do not overcook

7. Remove from the air fryer ; Let stand for 5 minutes. Carefully roll a knife over the sides of the Ramekins several times to loosen the cake.

8. Invert onto the dessert plates. Sprinkle with crushed candies.

9. Serve immediately.

Air Fryer Panko Breaded Chicken Parmesan with Marinara Sauce

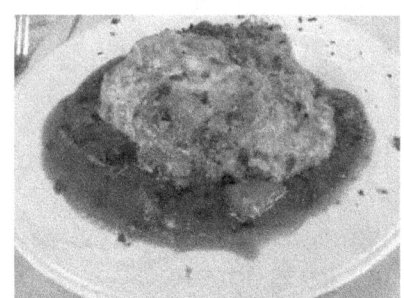

Air Fryer Panko Breaded Chicken Parmesan with Marinara Sauce is a quick and simple low-calorie, low-fat recipe with mozzarella cheese.

Ingredients

16 ounces of skinless chicken breast, cut in half for 4 breasts

1 cup panko breadcrumbs

1/2 cup grated Parmesan

1/2 cup grated mozzarella cheese

1/8 cup of egg whites

2 teaspoons Italian seasoning

salt and pepper

cooking spray

How to cook Air Fryer Panko Breaded Chicken Parmesan with Marinara Sauce

1. Preheat the fryer to 400.

2. Spray the basket with a cooking spray.

3. Slice the chicken breast in half to obtain 4 finer chicken breasts.

4. Place the chicken breast on a hard surface and pound them to make them flat.

5. Grate the Parmesan cheese.

6. Mix panko breadcrumbs, cheese and spices in a bowl big enough to dip the chicken breast. Stir to combine.

7. Put the egg whites in a bowl.

8. Dip the chicken into the egg whites and then the breadcrumb mixture.

9. Put in the air fryer. Sprinkle the top of the chicken with a cooking spray.

10. Cook for 7 minutes. Garnish each breast with marinara sauce and grated mozzarella cheese.

11. Cook for 3 minutes more or until cheese has melted.

Roasted broccoli with cheese sauce

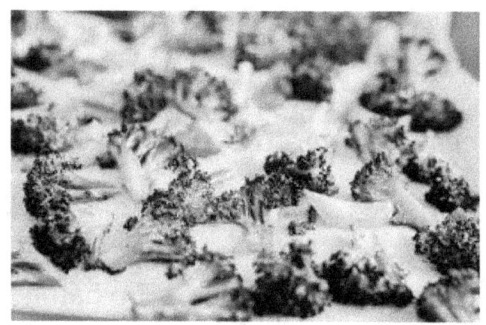

Ingredients

6 cups broccoli florets (about 12 ounces)

Cooking spray

10 tablespoons low-fat condensed milk

1 1/2 oz queso fresco (fresh Mexican cheese), crumbled (about 5 tbsp)

4 teaspoons aj amarillo paste

6 crackers

How to make Roasted broccoli with cheese sauce

1. Coat the broccoli florets well with cooking spray.

2. Place half of the broccoli in a frying basket and cook at 375 ° F until soft, 6 to 8 minutes.

3. Repeat the process with the remaining broccoli.

4. In the meantime, pour condensed milk, Queso Fresco, Ají Amarillo paste and salt into a blender; treat until smooth, about 45 seconds.

5. Put the sauce in a microwave-safe bowl. Microwave at maximum power for about 30 seconds.

6. Serve the cheese sauce with broccoli.

TSO chicken

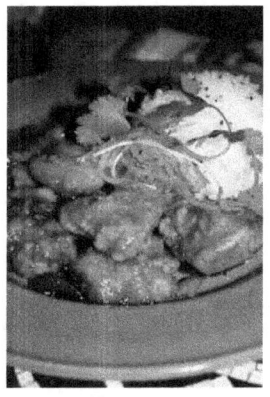

Ingredients

1 large egg

1 pound boned skinless chicken thighs,

1/3 cup plus 2 tbsp. Cornstarch,

1/4 teaspoon kosher salt

1/4 teaspoon ground pepper

7 tablespoons less cooked sodium broth

2 tablespoons soy sauce

4 peppers chopped and seeds thrown

1 tablespoon fresh ginger finely chopped

1 tablespoon garlic finely chopped

2 tablespoons chopped green onion, split

How to make TSO chicken

1. Beat the egg in a large bowl, add the chicken and coat well.

2. In another bowl, mix 1/3 cup cornstarch with salt and pepper.

3. Add the chicken to the cornstarch mixture with a fork and stir
with a spatula.

4. Place the chicken in an air fryer grid (or in a frying basket, in batches) leaving a small gap between the pieces.

5. Preheat the deep fryer to 400 ° F for 3 minutes.

6. Add the chicken; cook for 12 to 16 minutes, turn chicken halfway. Let it dry for 3 to 5 minutes. If the chicken is still moist on one side, fry for another 1 to 2 minutes.

7. Whisk the remaining 2 teaspoons of cornstarch with broth, soy sauce, ketchup, sugar and rice vinegar.

8. Heat the canola oil and the peppers in a large pan over medium heat, add ginger and garlic; cook for 30 minutes.

9. Whisk the cornstarch mixture; stir the mixture in the pan. Increase the fire to medium-high. When the sauce starts to bubble, add the chicken.

10. Stir; Cook until the sauce thickens and sticks well to the chicken, about 1 1/2 minutes.

11. Turn off the heat and add 1 tablespoon of green onion and sesame oil. Serve on a serving plate and garnish with remaining sesame seeds and green onions from a tablespoon.

Bourbon wings

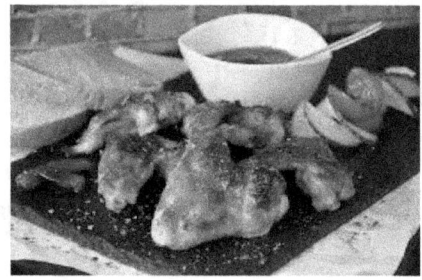

Ingredients

1/2 cup peach

1 tablespoon brown sugar

1 garlic clove chopped

1/4 teaspoon salt

2 tablespoons white vinegar

2 tablespoons bourbon

1 teaspoon cornstarch

1-1/2 teaspoons of water

2 pounds of chicken wings

How to cook Bourbon wings

1. Preheat the fryer to 400 °. Place peaches, brown sugar, garlic and salt in a food processor; process until smooth.

2. Put in a pan. Add vinegar and bourbon; bring to a boil. Lower the temperature; simmer, 4-6 minutes.

3. In a small bowl, mix corn starch and water until smooth.

4. Return to the boil and stir constantly. cook and stir for 1 to 2 minutes or until thickened.

5. Reserve 1/4 cup of sauce to serve.

6. Using a sharp knife, cut the two joints of each chicken wing.

7. Throw the wing tips. Spray the air fryer basket with a cooking spray.

8. If working in batches is needed, than place the wings in a single layer in the basket of the fryer.

9. Bake for 6 minutes, turn over and spread with canned mixture. Return to the deep fryer and cook until golden brown and the juice run clear, 6-8 minutes longer.

10. Remove and keep warm.

www.ingramcontent.com/pod-product-compliance
Lightning Source LLC
Chambersburg PA
CBHW072018070526
44583CB00015B/1527